Self-assessment
Clinical

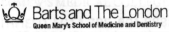

Related titles published in Mosby's Testing series include:

Clinical Dermatology
Clinical Infectious Disease
Clinical Medicine
Clinical Neurology
Clinical Surgery
Dermatology
Ear, Nose and Throat
Embryology, 2nd Edition
Endocrinology, 2nd Edition
Gastroenterology, 2nd Edition
Hematology
Human Histology
Human Anatomy
Hypertension

Infectious Diseases
Injury in Sport
Medicine:
  Vols 1–4
Obstetrics and Gynecology
Oral Medicine
Orthopaedics
Otolaryngology
Paediatrics
Pathology
Renal Disease
Rheumatology
Sexually Transmitted Diseases
Urology

Publisher: **Claire Hooper**

Development Editor: **Gina Almond**

Project Manager: **Jane Tozer** 25/4/97

Production: **Gudrun Hughes** M

Index: **Nina Boyd**

Cover Design: **Greg Smith**

Copyright © 1997 Times Mirror International Publishers Limited

Published in 1997 by Mosby-Wolfe, an imprint of Times Mirror International Publishers Limited

Printed by Vincenzo Bona

ISBN 0 7234 2591 4

For full details of all Times Mirror International Publishers Limited titles, please write to Times Mirror International Publishers Limited, Lynton House, 7–12 Tavistock Square, London WC1H 9LB, England.

A CIP catalogue record for this book is available from the British Library.

PREFACE

The increasing specialization within medicine in the United Kingdom presents particular challenges to the cardiologist or cardiovascular clinician practicing in the district general hospital. The cardiovascular clinician has to remain a general physician in order to recognize and understand the problems that are presenting which often reflect the relationship of the cardiovascular disease to other medical or psychosocial conditions. Therein lies an everlasting and intriguing challenge. Moreover, the role of the consultant in this setting is beginning to change. There are opportunities to develop a new style of consultant practice. The consultant of the next century will have a much more clearly defined responsibility for the local population both in terms of treatment and of disease prevention. This will involve an increased amount of devolved responsibility to nurse specialists and other health-care professionals; there will be different working relationships with general practitioners. These changed roles will be supported by the advances in information technology which will embrace information and advisory/expert systems developed for the practising clinician.

These diagnostic picture tests are from patients presenting to a district general hospital over a period of some years. Some of the problems presented here are common; others less so. The questions are intended to test knowledge at different levels of complexity; some invite a succinct answer, others are designed to produce a more discursive response. I hope this variety of questions and anticipated responses will serve to maintain the interest and stimulate the thought processes of the reader.

Non-invasive techniques continue to increase the potential to refine the clinical assessment of a patient presenting with a cardiovascular problem. These investigations should serve as a 'feedback loop' which informs and improves the clinical assessment at the bedside. The cardiologist, or cardiovascular clinician, occupies a privileged position since any patient undergoing investigations will have them performed within the cardiovascular department under a watchful eye. A knowledge of such patients passing through the department is valuable from a number of points of view; not only does it enable dissemination of information about the patient and the ability, if appropriate, to influence the subsequent management, but it is also a rich source of teaching material. I am grateful to the clinicians both within the hospital and in the primary care environment who requested these investigations. I am grateful also to the other health professionals working within our cardiovascular department. These include technicians, cardiographers, nurses and secretaries. Each one contributes something different and special. Their increasingly important roles are unfortunately not yet fully recognized.

ACKNOWLEDGEMENTS

To: Gillian

I am grateful to all my colleagues for the referral of their patients for an investigation or for an opinion. I thank the following for providing illustrations:

Dr Rachel Phillips   Professor Peter Ell
Dr David Grant   Dr A Rubin
Dr Suzanna Hardman   Dr Arthur Hollman
Dr D Hakhamaneshi

LIST OF ABBREVIATIONS

ACE	angiotensin-converting-enzyme
ARDS	adult respiratory distress syndrome
AV	atrioventricular
BP	blood pressure
CT	computerized tomography
ECG	electrocardiogram
ENT	ear nose and throat
FH	familial hypercholesterolemia
GP	general practitioner
ICU	intensive care unit
IV	intraventricular
JVP	jugular venous pulse
LA	left atrial
LDL	low-density lipoprotein
LSE	left sternal edge
LV	left ventricular
LVEDP	left ventricular end-diastolic pressure
LVP	left ventricular pressure
METs	metabolic equivalents of the task
MRI	magnetic resonance imaging
MUGA	multiple-gated acquisition
NMR	nuclear magnetic resonance
PA	postero-anterior (x-rays): pulmonary artery (pressures)
PAWP	pulmonary artery wedge pressure
PDA	patient ductus arteriosus
RV	right ventricle
SAM	systolic anterior movement
2-D	two-dimensional
TEE	transesophageal echocardiogram

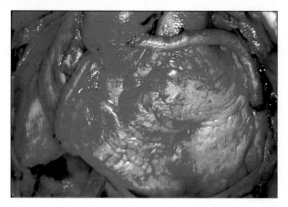

▲ 1

A surgeon has just taken this patient off bypass.

(a) What operation has been performed?
(b) What is the surgical mortality risk in a middle-aged man with stable symptoms?
(c) What is the duration of symptomatic benefit?

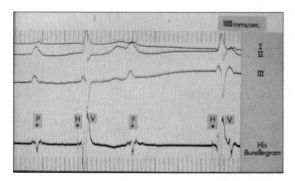

▲ 2

The recordings of the standard leads I, II, III together with the recording of the His bundle were obtained from a 36-year-old man who presented with tiredness.

(a) What is the rhythm?
(b) What do the H and V deflections represent?
(c) Is there any value in measuring the H–V interval and in what circumstances?

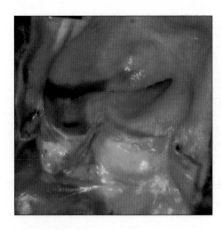

◀ 3
A picture of the aorta just above the aortic valve. This patient presented with chest pain and developed ventricular fibrillation in the accident and emergency department and could not be resuscitated.

(a) What is the likely cause of death?

(b) Why did the patient develop ventricular fibrillation?

(c) Are there any predisposing factors to this condition?

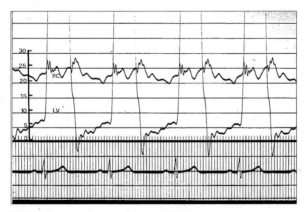

▲ 4
These pressures were recorded simultaneously with the electrocardiogram (ECG). The pulmonary artery wedge pressure (PAWP) or PC (pulmonary capillary) and the left ventricular pressures (LV) are measured in mmHg; the scale is shown.

(a) What are the two main abnormalities and how severe is the condition?

(b) Name two serious complications of this condition.

(c) What might the pulmonary artery pressure be?

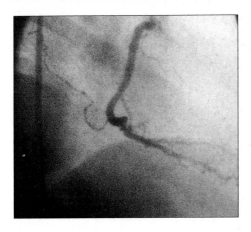

This view of a coronary arteriogram is taken in the right anterior oblique projection.
(a) Which coronary artery is it?
(b) Where does it run in the first part of its course?
(c) Name five of its main branches.

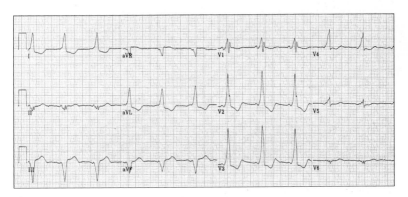

▲ 6
This 55-year-old man was admitted with lower sternal discomfort which started after a large meal. It was associated with shortness of breath. Physical examination was normal.
(a) What does the ECG show?
(b) How would you manage him?
(c) What other manifestations of his condition might he experience?

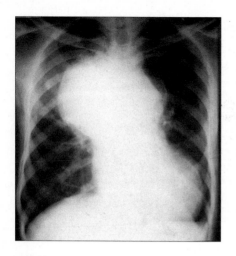

◀ 7

This 60-year-old man presented
with a five-month history of
dysphagia and shortness of breath.
On examination he was found to
have a heart murmur.
(a) What are the abnormalities in
   the chest X-ray?
(b) How do you account for
   these abnormalities, his
   dysphagia, and the murmur?
(c) What is the likely etiology?

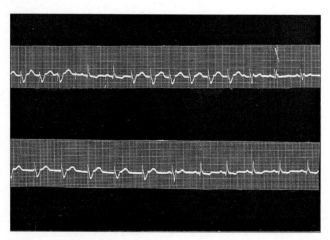

▲ 8

This 60-year-old man had a demand pacemaker implanted 4 years ago for intermittent
complete atrioventricular (AV) block and dizziness; he now presents with rather similar
symptoms.
(a) How do you account for the fact that he is in normal sinus rhythm without any
   pacing artefacts in the last part of the rhythm strip?
(b) Identify two abnormalities in the upper rhythm strip.
(c) What management for the patient do you suggest?

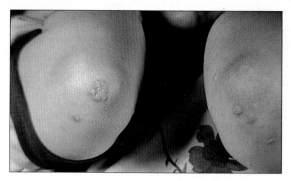

▲ 9

This woman presented with some upper epigastric pain. Initially admitted to exclude a myocardial infarct, on her second hospital day she developed these irritating lesions on her elbows.

(a) What might these lesions be?
(b) Where else may they be found?
(c) Why did she develop them?

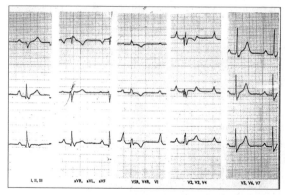

▲ 10

This 50-year-old woman with a long history of rather disabling recurrent palpitation and dizziness was known to have a heart murmur which was thought to be right-sided in origin. There was no clinical chamber hypertrophy. She was thought to be mildly cyanosed in the past but this had become more pronounced. The only abnormality on X-ray was that of a large heart.

(a) Identify four abnormalities on the ECG.
(b) Why does she have episodes of palpitation and become so unwell with them?
(c) What factors contribute to her cyanosis?

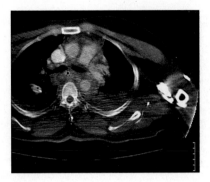

▲ 11

This 40 year-old-man was involved in a road-traffic accident. He suffered chest contusions as well as damage to his lower extremities; he was not wearing a seat belt. He was intubated because of respiratory distress. There was clinical evidence of pleural fluid at the left base. The contrast-enhanced CT scan of his thorax was reported as showing no obvious vascular disruption.

(a) Identify the main abnormalities on the scan.
(b) What particular type of vascular injury is likely to occur in this circumstance?
(c) If there were to be doubt about the vascular damage, what would be the definitive investigation and where should it be performed?

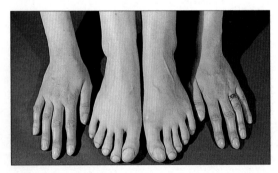

▲ 12

This 45-year-old woman was found to have a heart murmur at the age of 15, when her parents noticed that her legs and arm were often a different color compared with her friends. She was advised not to have any children. Her exercise tolerance is now quite limited by shortness of breath.

(a) What abnormalities do you note? How do you explain them?
(b) What complications of this condition might develop?
(c) Is there any treatment available?

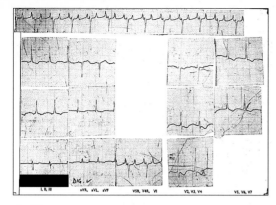

▲ 13

This 64-year-old man who was 30 hours postoperation had an emergency partial gastrectomy performed for a bleeding ulcer. He had been on digoxin for some years for heart failure but had not received any since before the operation. His immediate postoperative course had been satisfactory but he then, at 2 a.m., developed a tachycardia and his blood pressure dropped to 85/65/65 mmHg.

(a) What are the main abnormalities?
(b) What investigation would you ask for at this time of night?
(c) How would you treat the problem?

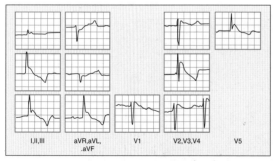

▲ 14

This 67-year-old woman had a history of mild angina for several years. She was brought into the accident and emergency department in a confused state by her daughter. She was on no medication and was found to have a pulse of 40/minute and a BP of 105/75/75 mmHg.

(a) What are the main abnormalities in the ECG?
(b) What other information would you like to confirm your diagnosis?
(c) How would you treat this woman?
(d) What possible complications might you expect?

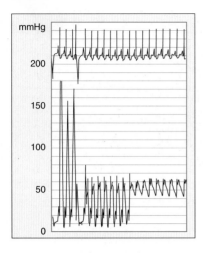

◀ **15**

This man was investigated by cardiac catheterization because of the symptom of syncope. He was found to have a heart murmur and an abnormal ECG.

The pressure tracing shows a withdrawal trace from the left ventricle into the aorta; in the first part of the withdrawal tracing there are a number of ectopic beats caused by the catheter tip irritating the ventricular wall.

(a) What is the main abnormality in this withdrawal tracing?

(b) What is the main differential diagnosis?

(c) How might the conditions be distinguished from each other?

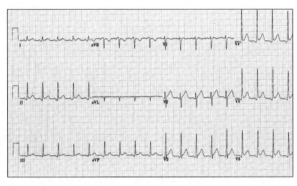

▲ **16**

This 28-year-old Nigerian man presented with some left submammary pain which was made worse when he was under stress at work. There were no abnormalities on physical examination.

(a) How would you report this ECG? The patient was in sinus rhythm.

(b) Could this ECG be within normal limits?

(c) What measures could you use to demonstrate the fact that the tracing is normal?

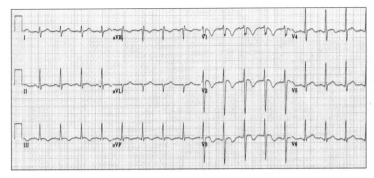

▲ 17

This 31-year-old man was admitted with some right-sided and central chest pain associated with dizziness. No abnormalities were found on examination apart from a slightly raised jugular venous pulse (JVP). He now presents with shortness of breath and more severe central chest discomfort. His BP has dropped to 95/70/70 mmHg.

(a) What does the ECG show?
(b) What is the likely diagnosis?
(c) How would you treat this man now?
(d) What would you do about his chest discomfort?

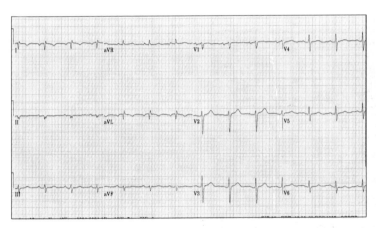

▲ 18

This 70-year-old woman developed some central chest discomfort. Her primary care practitioner was clinically suspicious of a myocardial infarction and requested an ECG.

(a) Name the two main abnormalities.
(b) What action might you take?

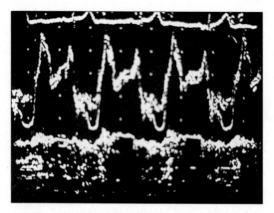

▲ 19

This 34-year-old woman presented with some left-sided chest discomfort, shortness of breath, and palpitation. On examination the heart was slightly irregular and there was a heart murmur that varied in intensity with posture.

(a) What abnormalities are present in the echocardiogram?
(b) What is the likely diagnosis and how do you explain the symptoms and signs?
(c) What is the natural history of the condition?

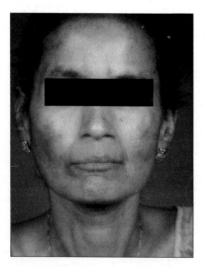

◀ 20

This 55-year-old woman who developed Raynaud's phenomenon 10 years ago is now getting progressively more short of breath on exertion.

(a) What is the most likely diagnosis?
(b) What other symptom might she have?
(c) Why is she short of breath and how might her heart be implicated?

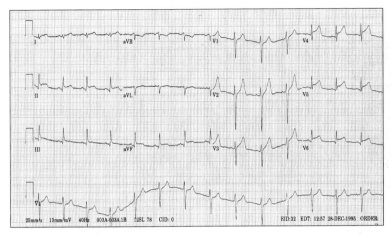

▲ 21

This 35-year-old man presented to his primary care practitioner with chest pain and was referred to the cardiac department for an ECG. He had no previous cardiac history.

(a) What are the main abnormalities?
(b) What is the main differential diagnosis?
(c) Is there any particular advice you would want to give this man once the diagnosis was confirmed?

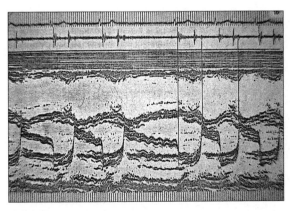

▲ 22

This man presented with a heart murmur and shortness of breath on exertion.

(a) What abnormalities are there on the echocardiogram?
(b) What is the most likely diagnosis and how severe is it?
(c) What do the two lines from the echocardiogram correspond to on the phonocardiogram and how do you account for the abnormalities?

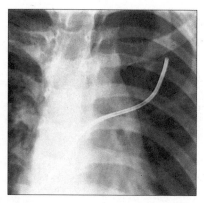

▲ 23

During a diagnostic cardiac catheterization the venous catheter which has been introduced via the femoral vein pursues the path displayed.

(a) What is the likely saturation of a blood sample taken from its tip?
(b) Name the vessel in which the tip of the catheter lies and describe the route the catheter took.
(c) What is the likely pressure in this vessel?

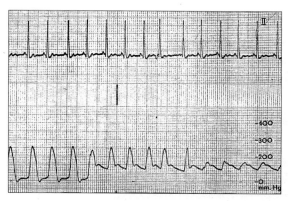

▲ 24

This withdrawal pressure tracing was recorded when the catheter was slowly drawn back from the left ventricle (starting on the left of the tracing) into the aorta. The ECG tracing at the top is to record the rhythm only. The patient had a heart murmur but was relatively asymptomatic.

(a) Describe the abnormality.
(b) Name two conditions that might produce this sort of withdrawal tracing.

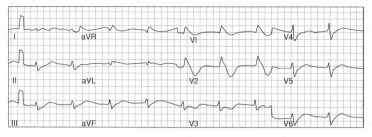

▲ 25

This 45-year-old woman was admitted semi-conscious. There were no localizing or lateralizing neurological signs. Her BP was 90/50 mmHg and she was peripherally constricted. Her heart rate was noted to be irregular and slow.

(a) What are the main abnormalities on the ECG?
(b) What is the likely cause of these abnormalities?
(c) If she were to collapse with a tachyarrhythmia, what is the likely mechanism of the arrhythmia?

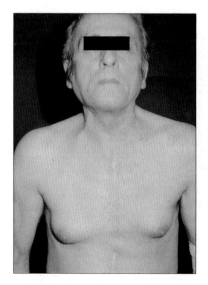

◀ 26

This man had a vein-bypass graft for angina some 5 years ago; he now has little angina but needs treatment to keep him out of heart failure.

(a) What abnormalities are there on inspection of his chest?
(b) Name two cardiac drugs that may cause this problem.
(c) Apart from the esthetic, are there any problems that may occur as a result of this condition?

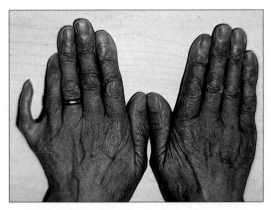

▲ 27

This 50-year-old woman presented with palpitations and a heart murmur. There was no heart failure and she was normotensive.

(a) What abnormality does she have in her hands?

(b) Why does she have a heart murmur?

(c) Is there a connection between these two problems? Is there an eponymous title for the condition and what is known of the etiology?

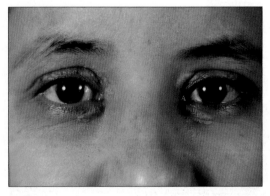

▲ 28

This 25-year-old woman from Kenya, of Indian parentage, was referred with these lesions around her eyes. She was otherwise asymptomatic.

(a) What is the composition of the lesions around her eyes?

(b) Are there any other abnormalities visible and what might their significance be?

(c) What measures should be taken after confirmation of the diagnosis?

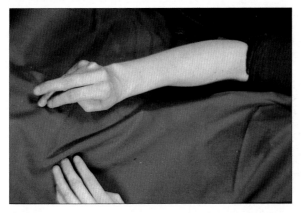

▲ 29

On inflating the sphygmomanometer to 120 mmHg the right hand of the patient rapidly adopted the displayed position.

(a) Why does the hand adopt this position?

(b) What associated abnormalities in the resting ECG might there be?

(c) Are there any described associations with this ECG abnormality?

▶ 30

This 24-year-old woman presented with a short history of shortness of breath, sweating, and some rather nonspecific chest discomfort. Her venous pressure was raised and increased with inspiration; her pulse was 110/minute and regular. Her BP was 110/70/70 mmHg and there was 30 mmHg of paradox.

(a) What does the X-ray show?

(b) How do you explain her hemodynamic state?

(c) What is the likely etiology?

(d) Why is the paradoxical pulse so called?

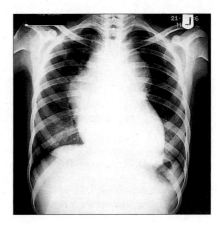

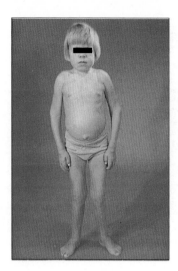

◀ 31

This 9-year-old boy has learning difficulties. He has had a hunched back and rather swollen knees for some years. His abdomen has always been protuberant. Recently a heart murmur has been noted.

(a) What condition does this young boy have?
(b) What are the other characteristics of this condition?
(c) Why does he have a heart murmur?

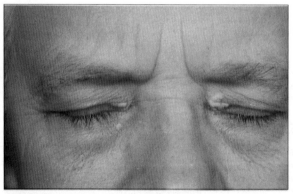

▲ 32

This 70-year-old woman was noted to have these lesions around her eyes some 10 years previously; they have not changed in size in the interval. She was otherwise well.

(a) What are the lesions?
(b) What is their significance in this age group?
(c) If she had an arcus would this be of any significance?

16

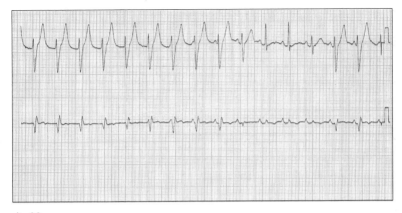

▲ 33

This 45-year-old man complained of palpitation. A 24-hour tape demonstrated rhythms which occurred in a cyclical fashion.

(a) What is the rhythm?

(b) What is the significance of this arrhythmia?

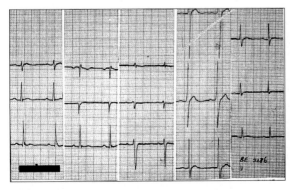

▲ 34

This 36-year-old man presents with shortness of breath and had a very abnormal chest X-ray.

(a) How would you report the ECG?

(b) How could the abnormalities be related to his chest X-ray?

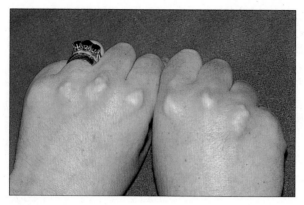

▲ 35

This 43-year-old lady presented with a 2-year history of discomfort and swelling in her ankles and wrists. She was otherwise asymptomatic. On examination she was normotensive.

(a) What are the abnormalities on her hands?
(b) How do the hand abnormalities relate to her arthropathy?
(c) What is the cellular abnormality that accounts for her problems?

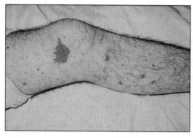 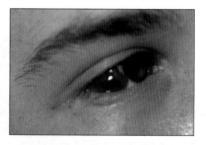

▲ 36, 37

This 20-year-old man presented with a fever and severe headache. His symptoms started 12 hours before admission. He had been previously well. His BP on admission was 85/70/70 mmHg; pulse was 120/minute. He rapidly became semi-comatosed. He had a skin rash over his trunk and more obviously over his legs. His eye was also abnormal.

(a) What condition do you think he has and how would you investigate and treat it?
(b) Why is the blood pressure so low and how would you manage it?
(c) Are there any other measures to be taken?

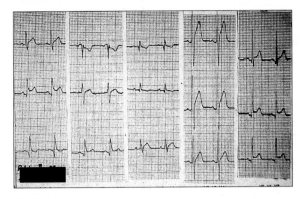

▲ 38

This 25-year-old man had a 3-day history of malaise and aches and pains together with a slight fever.

(a) What does the ECG show and what condition would you diagnose?
(b) Is there any other possibility that you would entertain?
(c) Is this always a benign condition? If not, what complications may occur?

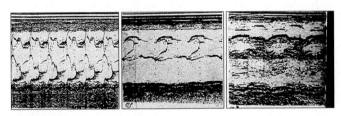

▲ 39

This M-mode echocardiogram was taken from a cyanosed neonate. The clinical diagnosis was that of congenital heart disease; there was no evidence of any lung disease. There are three views shown: the left is the mitral and tricuspid valves; the middle is the aortic valve and left atrium; the right is the pulmonary valve which is normal.

(a) What is the most striking abnormality?
(b) Why do you think the neonate is blue?
(c) Are there any other conditions associated with the lesion?

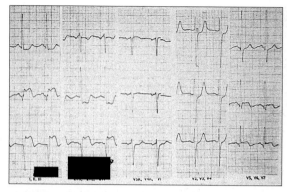

▲ 40

This 55-year-old man presented with severe epigastric pain; his BP was 80/60/60 mmHg and he had high venous pressure. He previously had a proven duodenal ulcer but was asymptomatic for a number of years.

(a) What are the abnormalities?
(b) How would you manage the persistent hypotension?
(c) How do you explain the phenomenon of ST-segment depression in this condition?

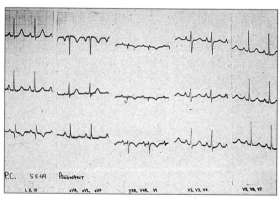

▲ 41

This 24-year-old woman was 32 weeks pregnant. She was short of breath and had palpitation, but had no chest discomfort. She had previously been in good health.

(a) How would you report the ECG?
(b) What are the main changes in the cardiovascular system in pregnancy and how long do they last?
(c) What happens to these changes at delivery?

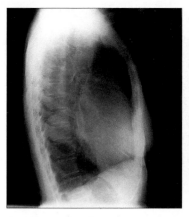
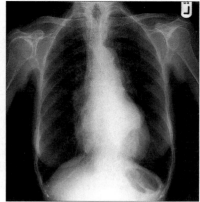

▲ **42**

This woman was referred with a soft-systolic murmur and found to have mild- aortic stenosis. Her chest X-ray was found to be abnormal. She was a life-long smoker.

(a) What are the main abnormalities in the posteroanterior (PA) and lateral chest X-ray?

(b) What is the likely etiology of the main abnormality?

(c) What treatment should be considered?

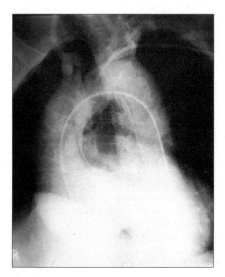

◀ **43**

This patient presented with central chest pain associated with sweating and shortness of breath. He looked unwell; his BP was 95/80/75 mmHg and pulse rate 120/minute. A murmur was heard over the precordium.

(a) What does the aortogram show (left anterior oblique view)?

(b) How do you think he should be managed?

(c) What conditions predispose to the development of this problem?

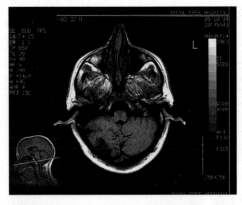

▲ 44

Magnetic resonance imaging (MRI) scan from a man who became unconscious following the treatment of his pulmonary embolism with heparin.
(a) What are the main abnormalities seen?
(b) What complication might ensue from the demonstrated abnormality?
(c) Why should an MRI scan be performed rather than other types of scan?

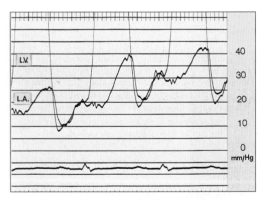

▲ 45

A pressure tracing of the left ventricle and left atrium ranges from 0 to 40 mmHg. There is also an ECG tracing. The paper speed is 50 mm/second. This patient has a long history of shortness of breath and has recently developed a heart murmur which has coincided with a deterioration in his symptoms.
(a) Identify three abnormalities in the tracings.
(b) What do you think the underlying problem is?
(c) How do you account for the heart murmur?

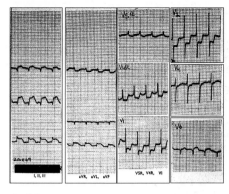

▲ 46

This 7-day-old neonate had severe respiratory problems related to heart failure. The child started to develop problems soon after birth but was not premature and had no heart murmurs. The mother had been ill with rather nonspecific symptoms for the last month of pregnancy.

(a) What does the ECG show?
(b) How do you account for the ECG and the heart failure at this age?
(c) What other causes of heart failure might you consider?

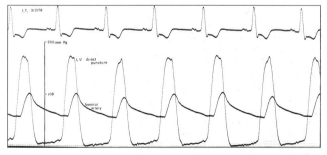

▲ 47

This tracing records the pressure in the left ventricle and the femoral artery simultaneously from a 60-year-old man who presented with shortness of breath on exertion and was found to have a heart murmur. The pressures are measured in mmHg and the scale is shown. There is also a simultaneously recorded ECG. The paper speed is 50 mm/second.

(a) Name four conditions that might produce this record.
(b) How might you grade the severity of the lesion on the basis of the information given?
(c) In a well person lying flat would the central aortic pressure usually be higher or lower than the femoral artery pressure?

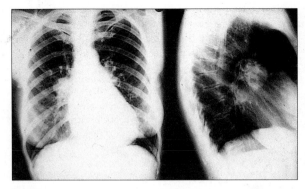

▲ 48

This patient was entirely asymptomatic. She had a routine medical X-ray for work which was reported as being abnormal.
(a) What do you think the abnormalities are?
(b) How might you confirm the diagnosis?
(c) What complications are associated with this problem?

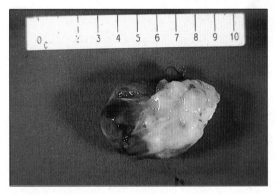

▲ 49

This mass was removed from the heart of a woman who presented with a stroke and was found to have a heart murmur.
(a) What do you think this mass is and where might it have been removed from?
(b) What other presentations are associated with this condition?
(c) How is the clinical suspicion of this condition best confirmed?

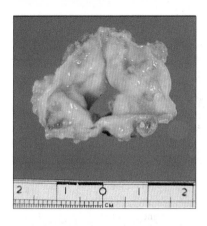

◄ 50

This valve was removed from a 55-year-old patient who was noted to have a heart murmur some 10 years previously.
(a) What valve is it?
(b) What murmur was the patient likely to have had?
(c) What might a chest X-ray have shown in this patient before the valve was replaced?

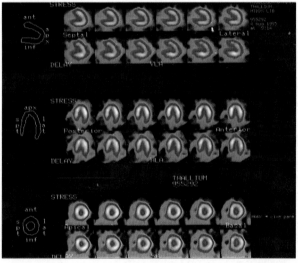

▲ 51

This 50-year-old woman presented with central chest discomfort which occurred on exertion and occasionally at other times as well. The clinician felt that this could be angina and sought confirmation of demonstrable ischemia in a thallium-stress test. The stress images in the lateral, anterior, and basal views are above the equivalent delayed images. The orientation is shown on the left-hand side.

(a) Why did the clinician use a thallium test rather than an exercise-stress test on the treadmill?
(b) What does the stress test show?
(c) What might the management for this patient be?

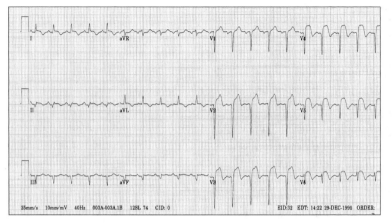

▲ 52

This 60-year-old man was admitted with central chest discomfort and shortness of breath.

(a) How would you report this ECG?

(b) Assuming his pain had now settled, his BP was 85/70/70 mmHg, and he was becoming oliguric, what would you do?

(c) If this man were to be risk-stratified what would be the outcome?

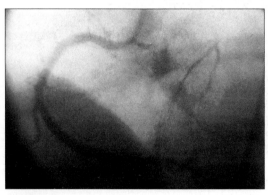

▲ 53

This right coronary arteriogram is taken in the left anterior oblique view. The patient had sustained an anterior infarct 4 years previously and was now suffering fairly severe angina on effort.

(a) Name five branches that are displayed in this arteriogram.

(b) Are there any abnormalities?

(c) What is the mortality risk from coronary arteriography?

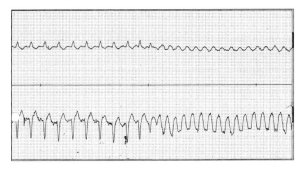

▲ 54

This 24-hour ambulatory tape recording was from a patient with a history of syncopal attacks. The tape had been put on and he was leaving the hospital when he collapsed.

(a) What does the displayed recording show?

(b) How should he be treated?

(c) What is this man's prognosis?

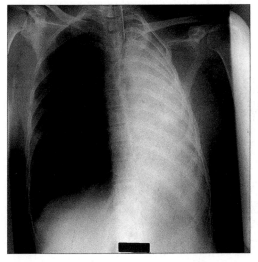

▲ 55

This woman of about 50 years of age was brought in collapsed to the accident and emergency department. She was resuscitated and intubated and when stable was brought to the ICU. The left side of her chest was not moving as well as the right.

(a) What are the main abnormalities on the X-ray?

(b) What is the likeliest cause of these abnormalities?

(c) What measures do you now take?

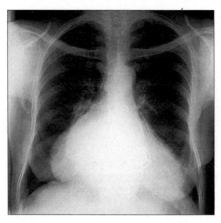

▲ 56

This 55-year-old woman who had surgery 5 years ago now presents with a high venous pressure, tender liver, and edema. Her lungs are clear.

(a) Identify four abnormalities in the X-ray.
(b) Are there any clues as to why she might have developed a high venous pressure and edema?
(c) What added sounds is she likely to have from the mitral prosthetic valve?

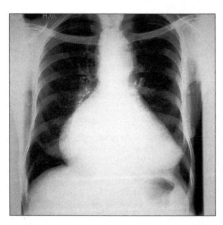

▲ 57

This X-ray is taken some 5 years after the one shown in **56**. The patient has started to lose weight and has dysphagia.

(a) Is there any difference in the X-rays?
(b) What causes of dysphagia can occur in patients with mitral valve disease?
(c) How might the diagnosis be pursued in this patient?

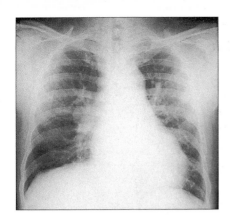

◀ 58

This man presented to Accident and Emergency after a fight outside a bar. He did not drink alcohol to excess. He was found to have a wide pulse pressure and a BP of 150/65/60 mmHg. There was a loud murmur, well heard, over the pulmonary and adjacent areas.

(a) How would you report this X-ray?
(b) How would you account for this murmur?
(c) What investigation would confirm this and what would it show?

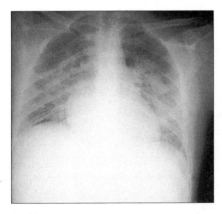

▲ 59

This 34-year-old man was admitted acutely ill with a BP of 80/65/65 mmHg, a pulse rate of 130/minute, and a respiratory rate of 25/minute. He had widespread crackles and wheezes, and a gallop rhythm. He was peripherally cool and afebrile, and was acidotic; his arterial blood gases showed a pH of 7.02. His ECG showed a sinus tachycardia; there was some minor ST-segment and T-wave flattening only. He had been a heavy drinker until 4 years previously. He had a chest infection which started about 5 days before admission. Prior to this he had been well and had a good exercise tolerance.

(a) What does the X-ray show?
(b) What is the likely cause for this problem?
(c) If he did not respond to diuretics, bicarbonate, digoxin, phlebotomy, or inotropes, is there anything else you might consider?

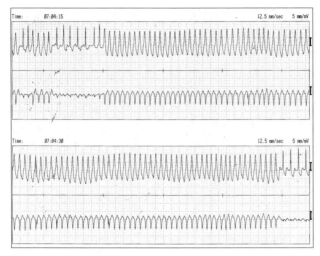

| Time: | 07:04:15 | | 12.5 mm/sec | 5 mm/mV |

| Time: | 07:04:30 | | 12.5 mm/sec | 5 mm/mV |

▲ 60

This 24-hour tape was recorded on a patient complaining of palpitation. There were no symptoms noted during the recording. There were no other cardiovascular problems. Two simultaneously recorded leads are displayed. The paper speed is 12.5 mm/second (half the usual paper speed) and the calibration is 5 mm/mV (half the normal calibration).

(a) What are the main abnormalities in the 24-hour tape?
(b) Can you be 100% certain about the mechanism of the arrhythmia?
(c) The patient was asymptomatic during the recording. Does this make a supraventricular arrhythmia more likely?

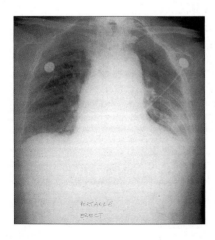

◀ 61

This 60-year-old man was admitted to the coronary care unit with central chest discomfort. In the past he had been treated for hypertension. The chest discomfort was associated with sweating and shortness of breath. On arrival his BP was 250/140/135 mmHg and his heart rate was 120/minute. His chest was clear.

(a) How would you interpret the X-ray?
(b) Are there any further investigations that you would request?
(c) What treatment would you introduce assuming that he was now free of pain?

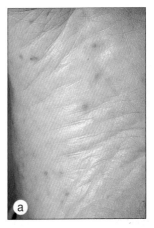

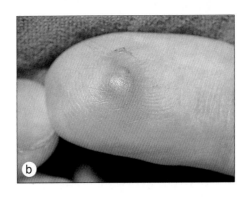

▲ 62

This 54-year-old man was admitted to hospital with nonspecific symptoms of an influenzal illness. He became very short of breath the day before admission. He was found to have a heart murmur which had not been previously recorded. He had a high swinging fever.

(a) What is the pathogenesis of the lesions on the sole of the foot (a)?
(b) What is the pathogenesis of the lesions on the finger (b)?
(c) What is the likely diagnosis?

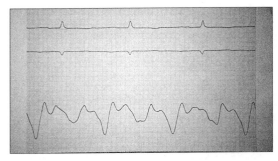

▲ 63

This tracing, recorded at 50 mm/second, is of two ECG leads together with a jugular venous pulse (JVP) recorded simultaneously. The patient had presented with a high venous pressure, a tender liver, and peripheral edema.

(a) Name the waves demonstrated in the recording and explain their genesis.
(b) Is there anything striking about the venous waveform?
(c) Suggest a possible diagnosis.

31

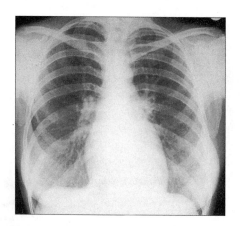

◀ **64**

This 40-year-old woman presented with increasing shortness of breath, orthopnea, and tiredness. She was normotensive and had a heart murmur.

(a) How would you report this X-ray?
(b) Why is she short of breath?
(c) Name five complications of her condition.

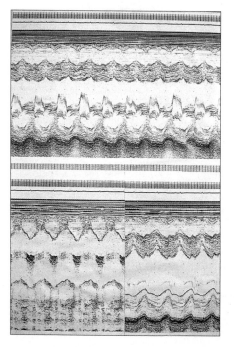

◀ **65**

This man in his 50s, who had rheumatic fever as a youth, had recently been short of breath; his heart was getting larger and the murmurs more pronounced.

(a) Name two abnormalities in the echocardiogram.
(b) Are you able to determine what murmurs he has?
(c) Can you explain the pattern of movement in the mitral valve?

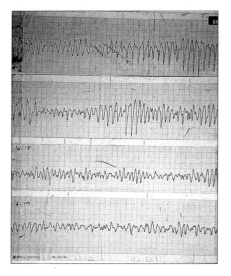

This patient who had collapsed in the street was brought in being resuscitated. There was no other history available.

(a) What rhythm is he in and how would you commence treatment?

(b) If he does not respond to your first measures, what might you do next?

(c) What conditions may predispose to this problem?

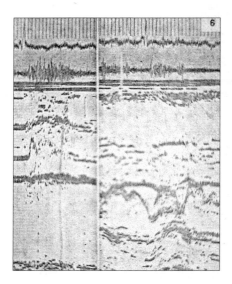

◀ 67

There are two views in this M-mode echocardiogram with a simultaneous phonocardiogram and ECG. The patient was mildly hypertensive and was referred by the primary care practitioner. A heart murmur was also commented upon.

(a) Name three abnormalities in the recording.

(b) Are you able to suggest a diagnosis?

(c) Is there any treatment that is required for this condition?

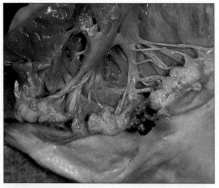

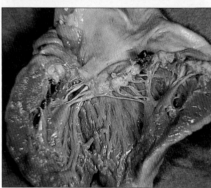

At autopsy the mitral valve of this patient was found to be abnormal. No clinical diagnosis had been made prior to death. She had presented with a confusional state and fever and died within 2 days of admission.

(a) What is the likely diagnosis?
(b) What is the prognosis for this condition in life?
(c) How is the diagnosis best made?
(d) How would you treat the condition and how would you know that the treatment was adequate?

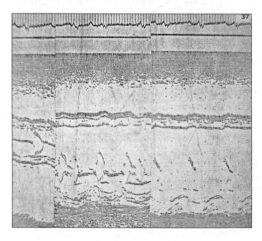

◄ 70

There are three views in this M-mode echocardiogram. The patient presented with a 2-year history of breathlessness on exertion, orthopnea, and ankle swelling. He was normotensive. There was a very soft mid-systolic murmur at the apex, an elevated JVP, and leg edema.

(a) What are the main abnormalities?
(b) What is the likely diagnosis?
(c) What is the possible etiology?

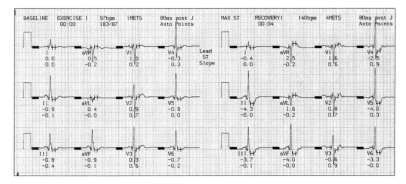

BASELINE	EXERCISE I 00:00	97bpm 183/87	1METS	80ms post J Auto Points		MAX ST	RECOVERY I 00:04	140bpm	4METS	80ms post J Auto Points

▲ 71

This 45-year-old woman had a history suggestive of angina. She was a smoker and there was a family history of premature death due to vascular disease. A diagnostic exercise test was performed. She was not on any drug therapy. She managed to achieve 4 METs (metabolic equivalents) and had to stop because of chest discomfort. Her blood pressure rose with exercise.

(a) How would you interpret the morphology of the ECG complexes?

(b) What is the sensitivity and specificity of this test in a patient such as this?

(c) Is her blood pressure response normal?

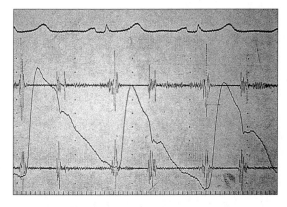

▲ 72

This is a simultaneous recording of the ECG, an indirect carotid artery tracing, and two phonocardiographic channels (apical area above, pulmonary area below). The patient had been found to have a heart murmur when pregnant but was asymptomatic.

(a) Name four abnormalities.

(b) What information can you learn about the severity of this condition?

(c) When would you be most concerned about her heart condition during pregnancy?

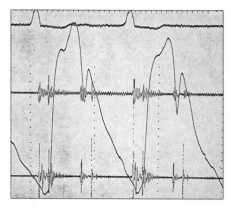

▲ 73

This is a simultaneous tracing of the ECG, an indirect carotid artery tracing and two phonocardiographic channels (pulmonary area above and mitral area below). The patient had heart surgery for valve trouble some 3 years previously and now has an improved exercise tolerance.

(a) Identify three abnormalities in the tracings.
(b) What type of valve surgery did the patient have?
(c) What complications are associated with these valves?

CATHETER DATA

Site	Pressure (mmHg)	Saturation (%)
Right atrium	6	70
Right ventricle	110/6	78
Pulmonary artery	25/10	80
Left ventricle	120/10	94
Aorta	120/80	88
Left atrium	10	98

▲ 74

The data presented above were obtained at cardiac catheterization. The patient was a 22-year-old man who had a heart murmur diagnosed at the age of 4 but had not been followed up. He is now slightly cyanosed and has an impaired exercise tolerance.

(a) Name three abnormalities.
(b) What is the likely diagnosis?
(c) Name a number of complications of this condition.

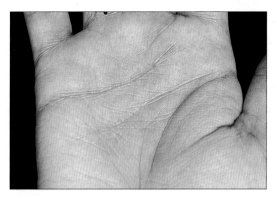

▲ 75

The palm of a man in his 50s is shown. He presented with an itchy rash over the extensor aspects of his forearm and irritation in both his palms. Both palms were discolored.

(a) What abnormality is demonstrated?
(b) What is the likely cause of this abnormality?
(c) How would you treat it?

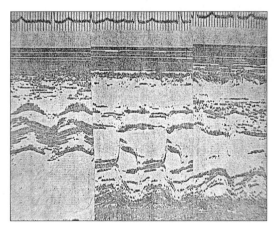

▲ 76

This 55-year-old patient had a history of rheumatic fever and was known to have a heart murmur.

(a) Identify the main abnormalities.
(b) What diagnosis seems likely?
(c) How severe is the problem?

CATHETER DATA

Site	Pressure (mmHg)	Saturation (%)
Right atrium	5	68
Right ventricle	45/5	70
Pulmonary artery	45/25	70
PA wedge	24	-
Left ventricle	125/23	98
Aorta	125/85	97

▲ 77

The data shown above were obtained from cardiac catheterization. The patient was a 33-year-old with increasing shortness of breath.
(a) Identify the abnormalities.
(b) What is the basis for the abnormalities?
(c) Suggest five possible etiologies.

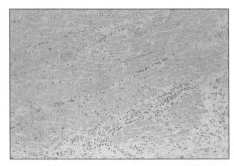
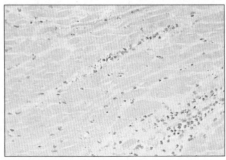

◄ 78, 79

These two histologic pictures of the myocardium of different magnification are from a patient who died suddenly while awaiting valve surgery.
(a) What is the abnormality seen?
(b) How might it relate to the patient's condition?
(c) How soon after this pathologic event can changes be demonstrated in the laboratory?

CATHETER DATA

Site	Pressure (mmHg)	Saturation (%)
Right atrium	3/0	70
Right ventricle	35/4	69
Pulmonary artery	35/15	85
PA wedge	9/5	-
Left ventricle	110/5	98
Aorta	110/80	98

▲ 80

The catheter data above were obtained from a 45-year-old man who was rather more short of breath over the past year than he had been previously. His primary care practitioner arranged an X-ray as a result of which he was referred to you.

(a) What did the chest X-ray show?

(b) On which chamber of the heart does the load fall in this condition?

(c) How should it be treated?

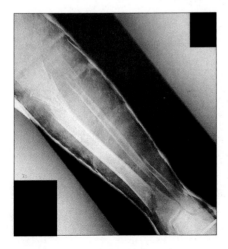

◀ 81

A 23-year-old man was involved in a road-traffic accident. There was no suggestion of any head injury. After fixation of some of the broken bones, he made good progress for 12 hours. He then became rather confused and aggressive and was given some analgesia. An hour later he had a cardiac arrest.

(a) What possible causes for the arrest would you consider?

(b) What other complications might you be on the alert for after the resuscitation?

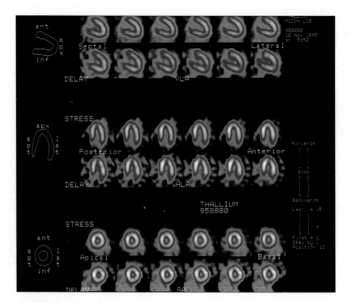

▲ 82

This thallium scan is from a 42-year-old woman who presented with chest pain which troubled her both on exertion and at rest.

(a) What are the particular advantages of thallium-stress testing over conventional exercise-stress testing on a treadmill?

(b) How would you interpret this scan?

(c) What are the main disadvantages of a thallium scan?

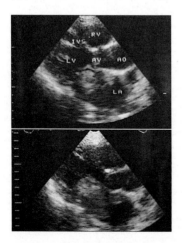

◄ 83

This 64-year-old patient presented with a transient stroke. The patient had been non-specifically unwell for a week before admission.

(a) How would you interpret the two-dimensional (2-D) echocardiogram?

(b) How does it relate to the presentation?

(c) What should further management entail?

(d) Are there any long-term problems that need be considered?

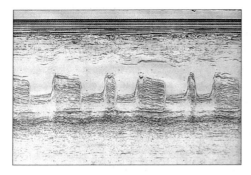

▲ 84

This 65-year-old patient was diagnosed as having mitral valve disease.

(a) How would you report this M-mode echocardiogram?

(b) What physical signs cause this condition to be confused with mitral valve disease?

(c) Name two limitations of M-mode echocardiography.

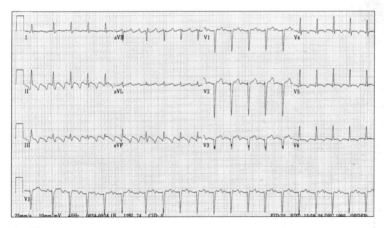

▲ 85

This ECG was taken on a male patient aged 57 who was complaining of palpitation. He had actually fainted on two occasions and felt like fainting on several others.

(a) What are the main abnormalities in the ECG?

(b) Why, in the context of a normal heart, is he tolerating this arrhythmia so badly?

(c) How might this arrhythmia be diagnosed at the bedside without an ECG?

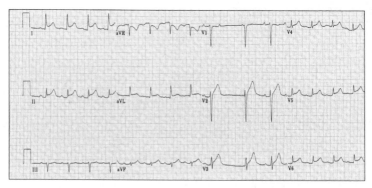

▲ 86

This ECG was taken on a 42-year-old woman who presented with a viral illness and central chest discomfort. Her venous pressure was slightly elevated and rose with inspiration.

(a) What are the main abnormalities?
(b) Is there any significance to her venous pressure?
(c) What other physical signs might you seek at the bedside?

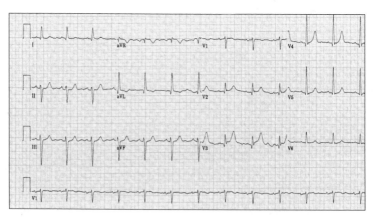

▲ 87

This ECG was taken on an 86-year-old man who presented with shortness of breath.

(a) What are the main abnormalities?
(b) If this man were to have a general anesthetic, are there any cardiac precautions you would like to take?
(c) What is the likely pathogenesis of his abnormal ECG?

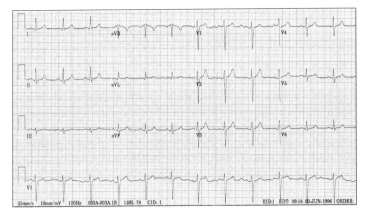

▲ 88

This 20-year-old man was admitted with chest pain. He had been complaining of tiredness for some weeks previously. He was a tall, thin, fit individual. Nothing abnormal was detected. His blood pressure was normal.

(a) How would you report the ECG?

(b) Does the ECG help in the making of a diagnosis in this instance?

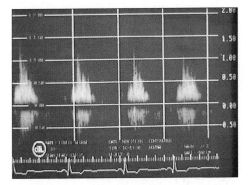

▲ 89

This continuous-wave Doppler study was performed from the suprasternal approach on a patient who had the clinical signs of aortic stenosis of moderate severity. This was presumed to be due to previous rheumatic fever. The patient had recently presented with mild heart failure. The ECG is shown below. The vertical axis represents flow in m/second.

(a) What is the advantage of the continuous-wave mode in this instance?

(b) What alternative to continuous-wave Doppler is there and what are its advantages?

(c) Can the severity of the valve lesion be estimated? If so, how severe is the problem with this patient?

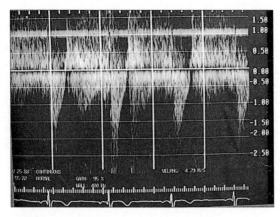

▲ 90

This continuous-wave Doppler, using the apical approach, was recorded from a patient with aortic valve disease.

(a) Can you comment on the significance of the waveforms?

(b) Can you quantify the severity of the lesions?

(c) Are there any other Doppler techniques that can improve the diagnostic yield from this investigation?

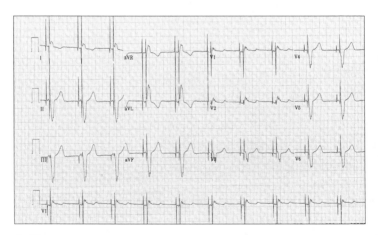

▲ 91

This 55-year-old patient had a pacemaker inserted following the discovery of complete AV block and the symptoms of syncope.

(a) What sort of pacemaker has been inserted?

(b) What is the advantage of this type of pacemaker?

(c) Why is this type of pacemaker not used in every patient?

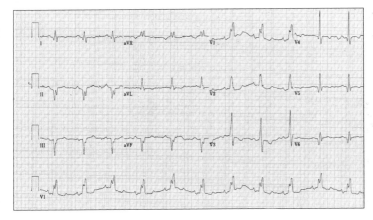

This 85-year-old man was admitted with a dizzy spell. He was on no drug therapy and previously had been well.

(a) What are the main abnormalities?

(b) What is the most likely cause of his dizzy spell?

(c) What is the preferred treatment?

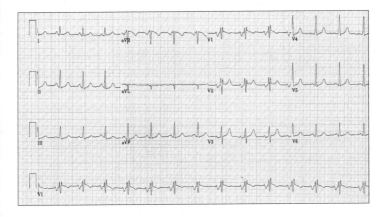

This 53-year-old woman was referred for an ECG because of shortness of breath. The ECG was reported as being within normal limits.

(a) Do you agree with the ECG report?

(b) What further investigations might be useful?

(c) Might treatment cause the ECG to change?

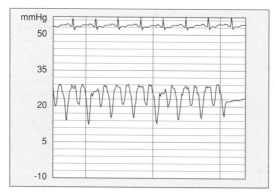

▲ 94

This 45-year-old woman presented with shortness of breath on exertion, swollen ankles, and distended abdomen. The venous pressure was elevated, her pulse was 90/minute, BP was 120/80/80 mmHg, and the chest was clear. She was comfortable lying down flat. There was no evidence of peripheral vascular disease. The illustration shows the right atrial pressure recording at cardiac catheterization with lead III of the electrocardiogram above.

(a) What are the main abnormalities?

(b) What is the most likely explanation for this waveform?

(c) Why does she not have orthopnea?

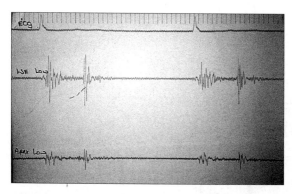

▲ 95

The simultaneous ECG and phonocardiogram were recorded from a woman who presented with shortness of breath.

(a) Name three abnormalities.

(b) Why might she be short of breath?

(c) What advantage does this type of recording have over the well-trained human ear?

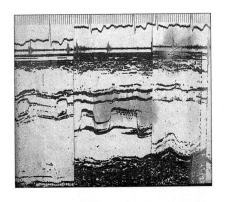

This 50-year-old woman who had a past history of rheumatic fever had increasing breathlessness in the last few months.

(a) Which chamber of the heart is enlarged? Why might it be large?
(b) Which valve is affected? Explain its abnormal movements.
(c) Is there any abnormality of movement of the left ventricle walls?

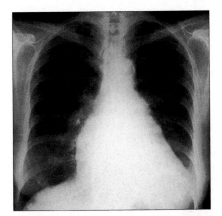

This 65-year-old woman presents with increasing tiredness, shortness of breath, and fatigue.

(a) Which chambers of the heart can you confidently predict are large?
(b) Can you make any inference about pressures in the heart from the plain chest X-ray?

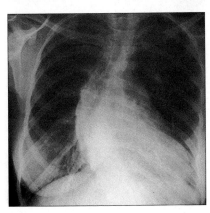

This patient was asymptomatic but was found to have a systolic murmur that had not previously been noted.

(a) How would you report the X-ray?
(b) Can you suggest the likely origin of her heart murmur?

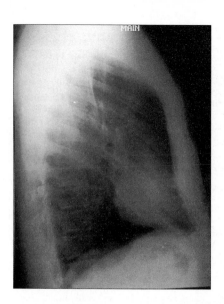

This 44-year-old man had an operation for a sternal depression for esthetic reasons. As a result of the sternal depression, heart disease may be mistakenly diagnosed in the following ways:

(a) Radiographically. Why?
(b) Clinically. How?
(c) Electrocardiographically. Why?

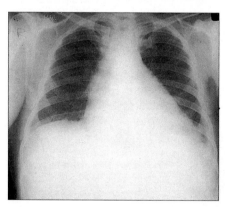

▲ 100

This 45-year-old Turkish man presented with a 3-week history of malaise, fever, cough, and shortness of breath. He was comfortable lying flat in bed; his BP was 110/70/70 mmHg; pulse was 110/minute; respiratory rate was 19/minute; venous pressure was elevated 6 cm above the sternal angle and increased with inspiration; temperature was 38.4°C.

(a) What does the X-ray show?
(b) How might you explain the physical signs?
(c) What other investigations might be useful?

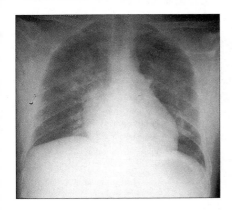

This previously fit 24-year-old presented with the rapid onset of shortness of breath over 4–5 hours. There was no preceding illness and no chest pain.
(a) What does the X-ray show?
(b) What conditions might lead to this presentation?
(c) How might this be treated?
(d) If the treatment specified does not work what condition might you consider?

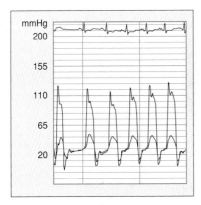

▲ 102
This 45-year-old woman presented with shortness of breath on exertion, swollen ankles, and distended abdomen. Her venous pressure was elevated, BP was 120/80/80 mmHg, and the chest clear; pulse was 90/minute and regular. She was comfortable lying down flat. The illustration shows the left and right ventricular recordings on the same pressure range.
(a) What abnormalities are displayed in the pressure recordings?
(b) How is this abnormality explained?
(c) Why was this patient short of breath?

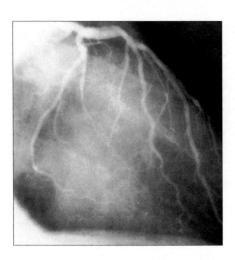

◄ 103

This is the right anterior oblique view of a coronary arteriogram of a patient.

(a) Which artery is it?

(b) Name five branches of the vessel.

(c) Does this vessel supply the conducting system of the heart? If so, does it supply it all or only part?

(d) Does this vessel supply any part of the interventricular septum? If so, which part?

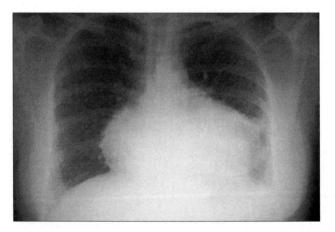

▲ 104

This 33-year-old woman presented with palpitation and some shortness of breath. She had suffered some upper respiratory tract symptoms which were now improving. She was known to have had a normal chest X-ray 6 months previously.

(a) How would you report the X-ray?

(b) What do you think is the most likely diagnosis?

(c) Are there any dangers associated with this condition?

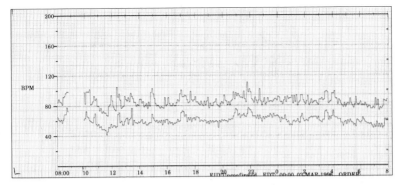

▲ 105

This recording is from an 82-year-old man in heart failure and atrial fibrillation. The heart-rate trend is displayed. The arrow indicates that the 24-hour tape recording started just before 10 a.m. The two lines represent the maximum and minimum heart rate in each 6-minute interval of the 24-hour recording.

(a) Why is this information useful in this patient?

(b) Would you expect this heart-rate distribution in the normal person?

(c) Should he be cardioverted?

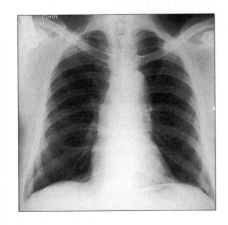

◀ 106

This 55-year-old man had a valve replacement with a prosthetic Starr–Edwards (SE) valve.

(a) Which valve has been replaced?

(b) What is the likely life of this sort of valve?

(c) What is the likely annual mortality from anticoagulation?

51

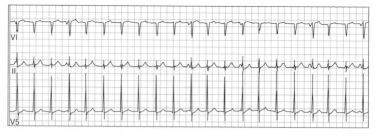

▲ 107

This 86-year-old man was experiencing palpitation. Following his ECG, which was interpreted as being sinus rhythm, a request was made for a 24-hour tape.

(a) Is the interpretation of the ECG correct?

(b) Would it be reasonable to perform a 24-hour tape and what extra information would it give?

(c) What is the cost of the 24-hour tape?

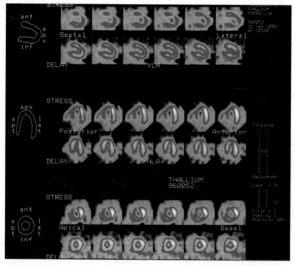

▲ 108

This thallium-stress test was performed on a 56-year-old woman who had suffered from chest pain for several years. The chest pain was difficult to characterize. When at home in the city it appeared to be related to exertion; when on vacation her pain was much reduced even on significant exertion.

(a) How would you interpret this thallium scan?

(b) Why is there a need for both a stress and delay picture?

(c) Why is there a difference in angina frequency related to the geographic locality?

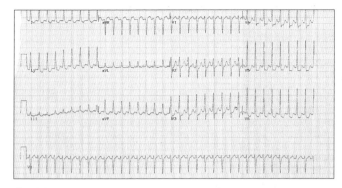

▲ 109

This 49-year-old man presented with a history of recurrent palpitation of sudden onset. There were no obvious precipitating factors. On physical examination he was found to be entirely normal.

(a) What does the ECG show?
(b) How might you best define the mechanism at the bedside and without the aid of an ECG?
(c) How should this arrhythmia be managed?

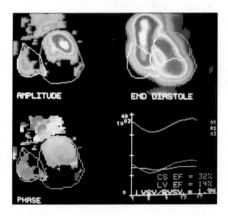

▲ 110

This 45-year-old man had sustained myocardial infarct some 3 years previously. He now presents with shortness of breath. His multiple-gated acquisition (MUGA) scan is shown.

(a) What comments would you make about the amplitude image?
(b) Is the phase image normal?
(c) The LV ejection fraction calculates out at 14%; what comments do you have?
(d) What other information is contained within this study; how does it help in the management of the patient?

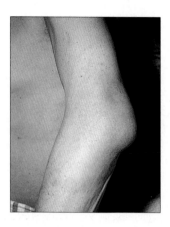

◀ **111**

This 64-year-old man was being treated for heart failure. He was in atrial fibrillation and on warfarin. He presented with a very uncomfortable elbow with overlying skin edema; it was hot to touch and painful. There were no other joints involved and there was no history of trauma.

(a) What is the likely diagnosis?
(b) How would you treat this man's condition?

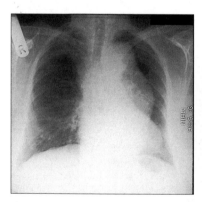 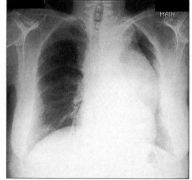

▲ **112, 113**

This 64-year-old woman presented with a history of occasional attacks of severe central chest discomfort radiating through to her back. Four years previously her ascending aorta had been replaced because of aneurysmal dilatation; at this time she also had severe aortic regurgitation which was cured by the operation on the ascending aorta without a need to replace the valve. X-ray **112** was taken in 1984, **113** was taken in 1988.

(a) What do these X-rays show?
(b) If surgery was advised, what would be the major morbidity risk; what sort of mortality risk might there be?
(c) What medical treatment might be helpful?
(d) What is the likely pathology underlying this condition?

Site	Pressure (mmHg)	Saturation (%)
Right atrium	a = 16, x = 8, v = 16, y = 5	70
Right ventricle	35/16	70
PA wedge	a = 17, x = 10, v = 16, y = 7	
Pulmonary artery	35/15	71
Left ventricle	120/17	98
Aorta	120/80	98

▲ 114

This 40-year-old woman presented with swollen ankles, distended abdomen, and shortness of breath on exertion. These symptoms had been getting progressively worse over 6 months. She had a normal blood pressure and a pulse rate of 95/minute. She was comfortable lying in bed with one pillow. Her venous pressure was raised. There were no murmurs. Her abdomen was swollen and the liver was enlarged and tender. Cardiac catheter studies showed the above.

(a) Name the main abnormalities.
(b) What is the likely cause of the problem?
(c) What is the best treatment?
(d) Why can she lie flat so easily?

Site	Pressure (mmHg)	Saturation (%)
SVC		68
Right atrium	a = 12, x = 0, v = 6, y = 4	70
Right ventricle	175/6	70
Pulmonary artery	10/4	71
Left atrium	a = 8, x = 3, v = 10, y = 1	99
Left ventricle	120/7	98
Aorta	120/80	98

▲ 115

This 35-year-old woman presented with a minor cerebrovascular accident but made a full recovery after several weeks. She was found to have a heart murmur.

(a) Name the main abnormalities.
(b) What physical signs might she have?
(c) How might one explain the initial presentation?
(d) If she were to become cyanosed on exertion, what might be the reason?

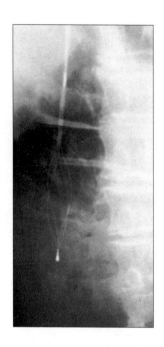

◀ 116
This patient was recovering from a myocardial infarction. The sleeve of an intravenous cannula had become sheared off from the hub and was sited in the right ventricle.
(a) What sort of catheter had been inserted?
(b) Why might there have been a need to insert this catheter?

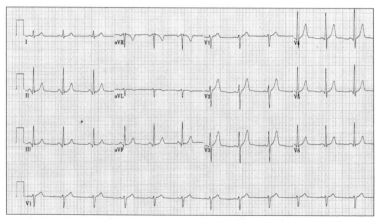

▲ 117
This 45-year-old patient had this routine preoperative ECG taken.
(a) How would you report this ECG?
(b) How valuable are routine preoperative ECGs?

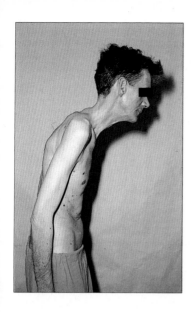

◀ 118

This 47-year-old man had suffered from lower back problems for many years. He had become increasingly short of breath over the preceding 5 years. He had also been noted to develop a heart murmur.

(a) What is the likely cause of his back problems?
(b) What is the likely cause of his heart murmur?
(c) Are there any characteristic ECG changes you might expect?

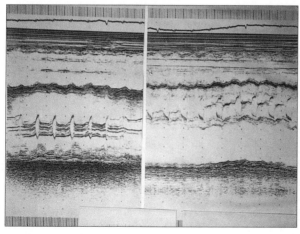

▲ 119

This 35-year-old man was admitted with severe shortness of breath, of recent onset. When admitted he was in quite severe heart failure and had a systolic murmur.

(a) Identify seven abnormalities in these two views.
(b) What sort of pathologic process may underlie this appearance?
(c) Why might he have a heart murmur?

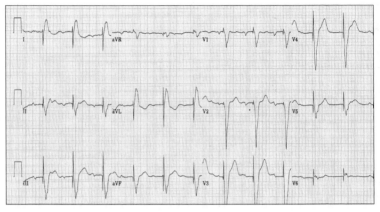

▲ 120

This 70-year-old man came into hospital feeling very weak. He was found to have a hemoglobin of 4.22 mmol/l.

(a) How would you report the ECG that was taken?

(b) Might he have an abnormality of his second sound?

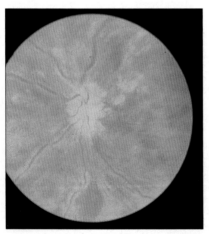

▲ 121

This optic fundus is from a patient who presented with sudden onset of blurred vision.

(a) What does the optic fundus show?

(b) What is the likely cause of these appearances?

(c) What are the predisposing factors to this condition?

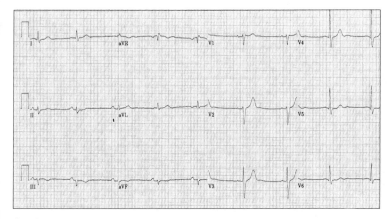

▲ 122

The ECG is from a man who was being treated for heart failure. He presented with increasing tiredness and lethargy. His thyroid function tests were normal and his heart failure seemed reasonably controlled.

(a) What does the ECG show?
(b) What treatment might you give him?
(c) Are there any foods that might help him?

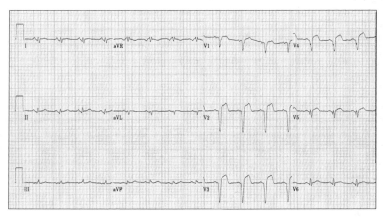

▲ 123

This 68-year-old patient was admitted to an orthopedic ward for a hip replacement. Two weeks prior to admission he had a severe attack of indigestion.

(a) What does the ECG show?
(b) What advice would you give to the orthopedic team?

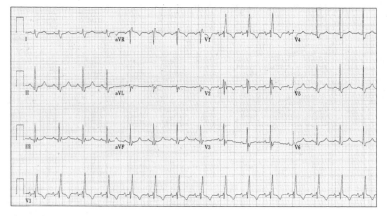

▲ 124

This 34-year-old rather overweight woman who was a bus driver had a Public Service Vehicle (PSV) licence. Physical examination was normal.
(a) How would you report this ECG?
(b) Can she continue to hold her PSV licence?

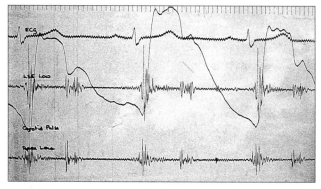

▲ 125

This is a simultaneous recording of the ECG, two photocardiographic channels (LSE, i.e. left sternal edge, low frequency and apex, low frequency), and the indirect carotid artery pulse. The recording speed is 50 mm/second. The patient, a 55-year-old woman, has been told that there is a heart problem. She is asymptomatic.
(a) Can you identify three abnormalities?
(b) Can you suggest a possible diagnosis?
(c) Is there any other feature that you might expect to find if this patient's problem were a severe one?

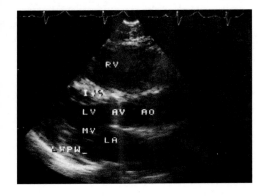

This 55-year-old woman presented with an atrial-septal defect. The chambers are labeled.

(a) What abnormalities might be found in the 2-D echocardiogram?

(b) Why is this a superior investigation to the M-mode?

(c) Is there any major limitation to the 2-D as opposed to the M-mode?

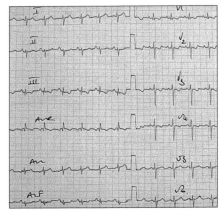

▲ 127

This 25-year-old woman presented with a history of two episodes of syncope on exertion. She was otherwise well. Physical examination was normal apart from a very short and soft systolic murmur at the left sternal edge and a loud second component of the second sound.

(a) How would you report this ECG?

(b) What information would you like to obtain from the chest X-ray?

(c) What other information would you particularly like to obtain from her?

(d) What information might be available if you were to perform cardiac catheterization?

Site	Pressure (mmHg)	Saturation (%)
SVC	—	69
IVC	—	71
Right atrium	a = 12, x = 4, v = 6, y = 4	70
Right ventricle	125/10	70
Pulmonary artery	125/85	71
PA wedge	a = 10, x = 5, v = 8, y = 3	
Left ventricle	120/7	98
Aorta	120/80	98

▲ 128

The catheter data shown above were obtained from a young woman who presented with shortness of breath and syncope on exertion.

(a) Name three abnormalities.

(b) What diagnosis might you consider?

(c) What treatment is available for this condition?

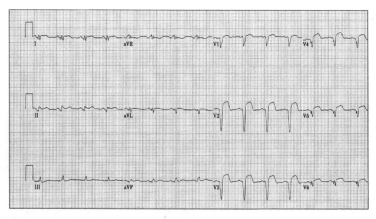

▲ 129

This 60-year-old man presented with severe chest pain radiating to his throat.

(a) What is the likely diagnosis?

(b) Could treatment cause the ECG to revert to normal?

(c) Are there any other investigations one might contemplate?

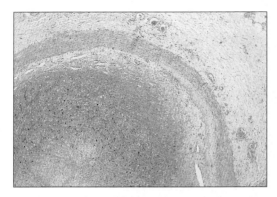

▲ 130

This histologic picture was taken from the coronary artery of a patient who had a history of angina for 3 years. He had collapsed and died while watching a football game.

(a) What does the picture show?
(b) What role does this play in the sudden death of this patient?
(c) Can this process be influenced to the patient's benefit?

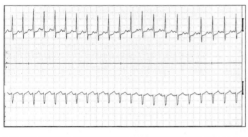

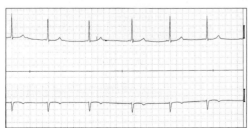

◀ 131

This 24-hour tape was recorded on a patient who complained of recurrent palpitation associated with dizziness. The tape used two leads; the top is a V5 equivalent and the bottom a V1 equivalent. The calibration is indicated to the right of the recording.

(a) What do the two recordings show?
(b) What measures might you advise the patient to take in order to terminate future attacks?
(c) What drug therapy might you use in this setting if necessary?

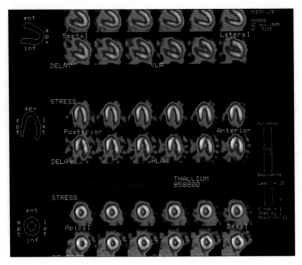

▲ 132

This woman presented with chest pain of several years' duration. An exercise-stress test showed ST-segment depression in the anterolateral leads but was not associated with chest pain. She had an adenosine-stress test performed.

(a) How would you interpret the result?
(b) Why is adenosine used and what is its mechanism?
(c) What is the specificity and sensitivity of this investigation compared with the conventional exercise test?

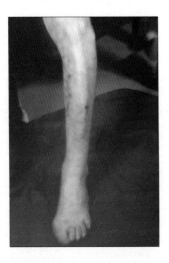

◄ 133

This 65-year-old woman presents with pneumonia and is found to have a heart murmur.

(a) What condition does she have?
(b) How might her heart problem be related to this condition?
(c) Are there any other heart problems associated with her condition?

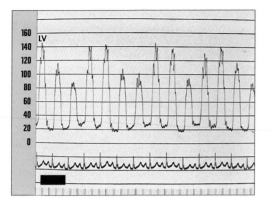

This patient presented 12
hours previously with
severe central chest pain.
The LVP (left ventricular
pressure) is measured in
mmHg and the scale is on
the left.

(a) Name two
abnormalities.

(b) What is the most
likely explanation of
his chest pain?

(c) Explain anatomically
how this condition
can occur.

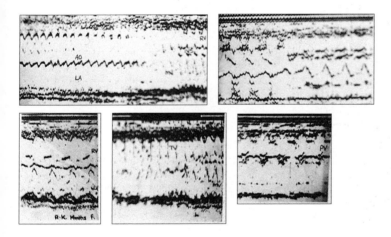

▲ 135

This M-mode echocardiogram was taken from a 3-month-old cyanosed child. A heart
murmur had been heard at birth and there was some cyanosis noted at this time, which
worsened over the next few weeks. The chambers of the heart are labeled.

(a) Are all the valves present?

(b) Is there any abnormal relationship between the aorta and the rest of the heart?

(c) What is the diagnosis?

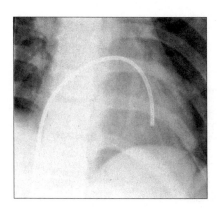

◀ 136
This patient with pulmonary stenosis was being catheterized from the right femoral vein. The blood drawn from the catheter in this site had a saturation of 97% and the pressure was 100/7 mmHg.
(a) Where is the tip of the catheter sited?
(b) How do you explain these findings?
(c) In what proportion of normal people is this maneuver possible?

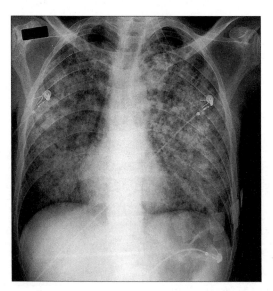

▲ 137
This 45-year-old patient was admitted to hospital extremely short of breath, and with a tachycardia of 140/minute and bilateral crackles. His BP was 85/65/65 mmHg. His chest X-ray is shown.
(a) What does the X-ray show?
(b) What is the most likely diagnosis?
(c) Why is he hypotensive and tachycardic?

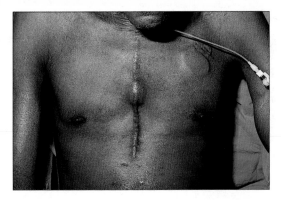

▲ **138**
This patient had an aortic valve replacement with a biological valve 8 years previously. Six months ago the valve had to be replaced because of degenerative changes leading to severe aortic regurgitation. At the second operation his aortic root had become very dilated and part of it had to be replaced. He now presents with a swinging fever, a continuous murmur at the base of the heart, and a wide pulse pressure. The lesion over his sternal wound slowly grows in size over a few days and becomes markedly pulsatile.
(a) How might you explain the enlarging lesion over his sternum?
(b) How might you explain the continuous murmur?
(c) Infective endocarditis would be the most likely unifying diagnosis. Is there any other diagnosis that might be considered?

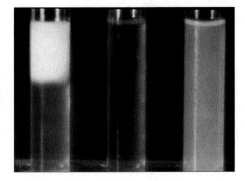

◀ **139**
What is the likely lipid abnormality in the patient whose tube is on the
(a) Left?
(b) Middle?
(c) Right?

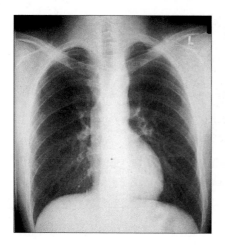

This 35-year-old asymptomatic man had applied for life insurance. He was found to have a BP of 150/95/95 mmHg. Otherwise, physical examination was thought to be normal.

(a) How would you report the X-ray?
(b) Are there likely to be any associated abnormalities?
(c) What might the optic fundi show?
(d) What might happen if you exercise him?

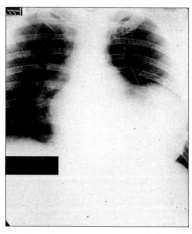

▲ 141

This patient presents with tiredness and shortness of breath.

(a) What is the main abnormality and what is it due to?
(b) Name four complications of this abnormality.
(c) Name three means by which the diagnosis could be confirmed.

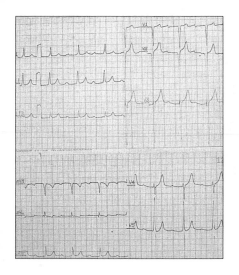

◀ 142

This 40-year-old man had developed mild aortic regurgitation 15 years previously. Over the ensuing years his regurgitation became progressively worse.

(a) Name two abnormalities.
(b) Can you suggest an etiology for his aortic regurgitation?
(c) Can you give an explanation in pathologic terms for your suggestion?
(d) What other clinical features might he have?
(e) Is there any predisposition to this condition?

Site	Pressure (mmHg)	Saturation (%)
Left ventricle	150/5	84
Aorta	150/85	88
Left atrium	12/5	93
Pulmonary artery	12/5	57
Right ventricle	14/0	54
Right atrium	14/8	54
Inferior vena cava		52
Superior vena cava		59

▲ 143

This 52-year-old man presented with shortness of breath on exertion. He felt generally unwell with many nonspecific symptoms. He also had some stomach distension but no bowel disturbance. Physical examination was unremarkable apart from a raised JVP. His catheter study is shown above.

(a) What are the main abnormalities in the recorded pressures?
(b) What are the main abnormalities in the saturations recorded?
(c) What is the likeliest diagnosis?

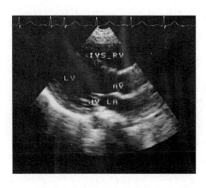

◀ 144

This 15-year-old boy presented with a high fever and a systolic murmur. The possibility of endocarditis on the mitral valve was raised on the request form.

(a) How would you report this echocardiogram?
(b) How would you advise about the possibility of endocarditis?

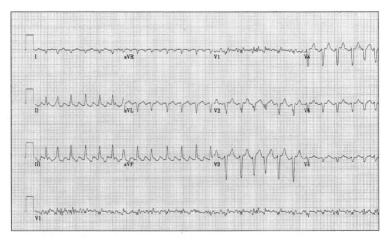

▲ 145

This 70-year-old man was admitted with heart failure. He was on no treatment.

(a) How would you report the ECG?
(b) What treatment for his heart failure does he need?
(c) Is any other treatment required?

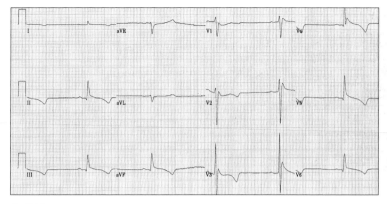

▲ 146

This 66-year-old patient was admitted from the accident and emergency department having been found collapsed at home. There was no other history available.

(a) Name three abnormalities.
(b) What is the most likely diagnosis?
(c) Give three reasons why the circulating volume of this patient might be low.

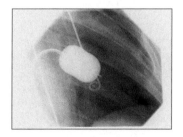

▲ 147

This woman had a long history of progressively worsening shortness of breath on exertion and had recently developed orthopnea and paroxysmal nocturnal dyspnea. She was found to have a heart murmur.

(a) What instrument is being used to address her underlying problem?
(b) How is the instrument sited in this chamber and what is the chamber?
(c) Are there any complications that you might anticipate?

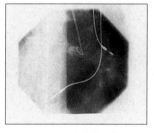

▲ 148

This patient was found to have a heart murmur. She had had a pacemaker inserted a few years previously when the murmur had not been noted. She has a pig-tailed catheter in her aorta.

(a) Can you determine the type of pacemaker?
(b) Can you define any valve problem?
(c) Is there any way that the conduction problem and the valve disease can be linked?

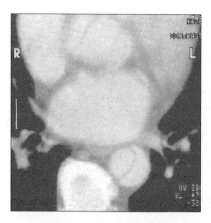

◀ 149

This CT scan is taken at the level of the heart. The patient presented with chest pain and the ECG showed pronounced ischemia.
(a) Identify the main abnormality.
(b) What is shown lying posterior to the ascending aorta?
(c) What are the two symmetrically placed structures which join the structure identified in (b)?
(d) What is the rounded structure lying on the left posterolateral aspect of the structure identified in (b)?

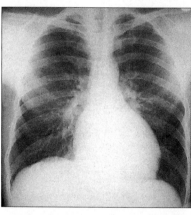

◀ 150

This 35-year-old homosexual man presented with fatigue and shortness of breath. He had a persistent sinus tachycardia and a normal blood pressure. He was apyrexial and had no heart murmurs. He had some crackles at both bases.
(a) What does the X-ray show?
(b) How might it relate to his symptoms?
(c) In what way could his sexuality have played a part in causing his heart problem?

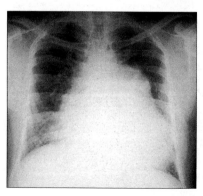

◀ 151

This 35-year-old man from Sri Lanka presented with shortness of breath and was found to have a loud heart murmur.
(a) What are the main abnormalities?
(b) What is the likely diagnosis?
(c) How do you think that this might be best treated?
(d) Are there any contraindications to the best form of treatment?

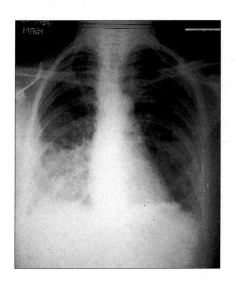

This 65-year-old woman was admitted to the ICU with progressively worsening shortness of breath. She was transferred from a medical ward where she was being treated for a stroke from which she was making a slow recovery. She was being fed with a nasogastric tube.

(a) Identify the main abnormalities.
(b) What is the likely cause of these changes?
(c) How is she best treated?

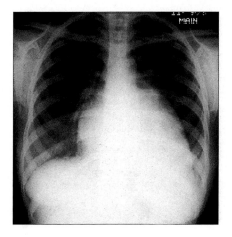

This 34-year-old woman presented with increasing shortness of breath, palpitation, and ankle swelling. She was found to be in mild heart failure and to have some heart murmurs.

(a) Name three abnormalities.
(b) Which chamber of the heart is the main culprit as regards her cardiomegaly?
(c) What is the likely etiology of her problems?
(d) What choice in the type of valve replacement is there?

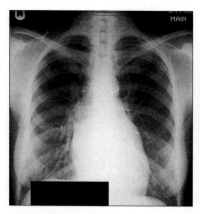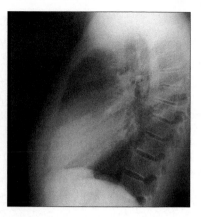

▲ 154, 155

These lateral and PA X-rays were taken from a patient who presented 9 months previously with a history of shortness of breath and was found to be in atrial fibrillation and to have a heart murmur. She now presents with the sudden onset of a left-sided weakness.

(a) How would you report the PA film?
(b) How would you report the lateral film?
(c) Is there any gut problem that may be associated with this patient's problems?
(d) How would you now manage her stroke?

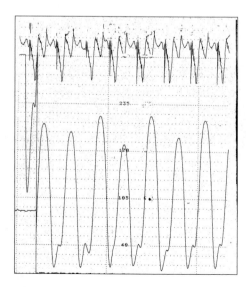

◀ 156

This pressure recording from the left ventricle was taken from a patient who presented with a heart murmur and was diagnosed as having aortic stenosis.

(a) What are the main abnormalities?
(b) Is there any significance you can attach to the waveform?
(c) What is her prognosis without surgery?

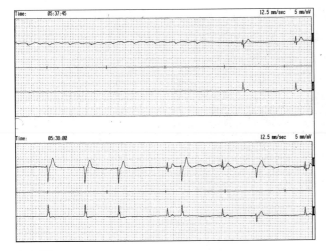

▲ 157

This 75-year-old woman presented with numerous episodes of dizziness and syncope. She had been witnessed to go pale, become absent minded, then briefly lapse into unconsciousness. She had sometimes been incontinent and had clonic movements of her arms during an episode. Her 24-hour tape was associated with several such episodes; it is displayed at 12.5 mm/second, the calibration is at 5 mm/mV. The top lead is a V5 equivalent, the bottom a V1 equivalent.

(a) This rhythm was recorded while she was asleep. How would you report the rhythm abnormality?

(b) How would you treat this arrhythmia?

(c) As this symptomatology has lasted some months is there any urgency to treat?

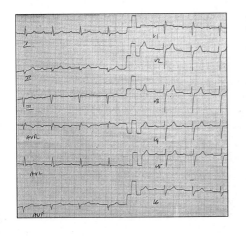

◀ 158

This 76-year-old woman with hypertension presents with dizzy spells.

(a) Name three anomalies.

(b) What is the likely cause of her dizzy spells?

(c) How would you treat her?

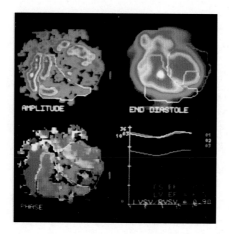

◀ 159

This patient suffered severe shortness of breath which was sometimes associated with exertional chest discomfort. His symptoms were limiting in spite of drug therapy.

(a) What radio-isotope study has been performed?
(b) Can you explain the principle of it?
(c) Are there any conditions of the patient which make this study virtually impossible?
(d) In which circumstances is this investigation particularly useful?
(e) What does this scan show?

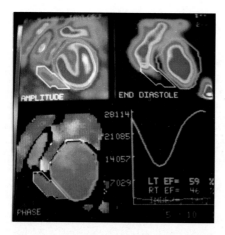

◀ 160

This MUGA scan was performed on a patient complaining of increasing shortness of breath on exertion.

(a) Explain the terms 'phase' and 'amplitude' which are the titles for the two pictures on the left.
(b) The ejection fraction is calculated as 59%. Is this normal?
(c) What comments do you have about this study?

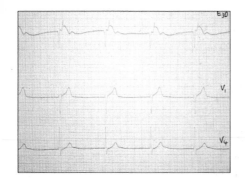

This patient presented with a slow regular bradycardia. These three leads were simultaneously recorded; the top recording is from an esophageal lead at 30 cm from the mouth. The middle tracing is V1 and the lower V4.

(a) What is the rhythm?
(b) Could you diagnose this clinically at the bedside?
(c) What is the virtue of the esophageal lead?

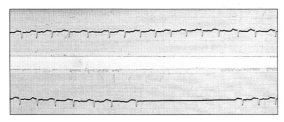

▲ 162

This continuous-rhythm strip of lead I was taken from a patient who was complaining of dizzy spells and who had collapsed on one occasion.

(a) What rhythms are present?
(b) How might you treat this patient?
(c) What sort of disease process is present?

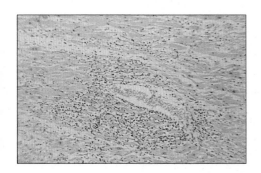

◀ 163

This 25-year-old woman had collapsed at home. There was no past history of heart disease.

(a) What abnormalities are present in this histologic section of her heart?
(b) What is the likely diagnosis?
(c) How common is this problem?
(d) What advice can be given to patients with this condition to reduce the risk of death?

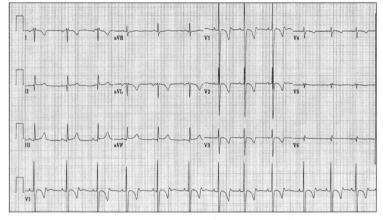

▲ 164

This ECG was requested by the ENT department prior to the patient having an operation. The patient had no cardiovascular symptoms and had normal blood pressure.

(a) How would you report the ECG?

(b) How might you relate the ECG findings to the requesting source?

(c) What is the pathophysiology of the condition?

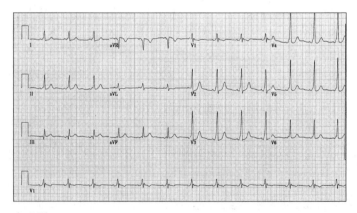

▲ 165

This 35-year-old man presented with two episodes of syncope. He had no cardiovascular symptoms and there were no abnormalities on examination. His BP was 120/80/80 mmHg. He had initially been referred to a neurologist who had performed an ECG.

(a) Are you happy to accept that this ECG is normal?

(b) What is the likeliest mechanism of his episodes of syncope?

(c) What further investigations might you contemplate?

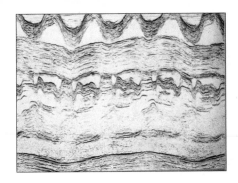

◀ 166
This 50-year-old patient presented with angina of effort and dizziness after exertion. A systolic murmur was found with a normal second sound.

(a) Name four abnormalities in the recording.
(b) What is the likely diagnosis?
(c) Are the symptoms described typical or atypical? Explain your answer.
(d) How might the patient die and how might it be prevented?
(e) Should the family be screened?

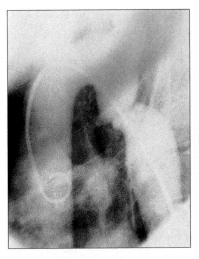
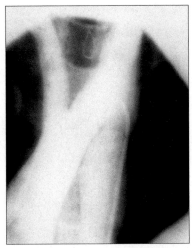

▲ 167, 168
This patient presents with the signs of a bicuspid aortic valve and mild hypertension. An angiogram is performed.

(a) In the lateral and PA projections of the angiogram, can you determine what condition the patient has?
(b) Why is surgery usually recommended?
(c) What physical signs is the patient likely to have?
(d) What are the other associated features of this condition?
(e) What is the particular risk of surgery in this condition?

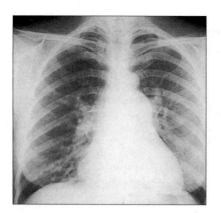

◄ 169

This 65-year-old woman had had a murmur for a number of years. She had noted increasing shortness of breath in the past year or two.

(a) What are the main abnormalities?
(b) What is the likely diagnosis?
(c) How severe is the lesion?
(d) How might you determine the advisability of surgery?

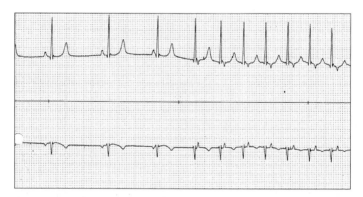

▲ 170

This 55-year-old woman presented with symptoms of palpitation which had been present for about 3 years. There were no obvious precipitating factors. The palpitations were associated with some light-headed feeling but no syncope. Physical examination was entirely normal and her resting ECG was normal. During the 24-hour tape recording she experienced some palpitation. In the recording there were two leads recorded simultaneously, the top one reflecting a V5 equivalent and the bottom one a V1 equivalent.

(a) The tape was reported as showing sinus rhythm with runs of supraventricular tachycardia. Do you agree with this assessment?
(b) Might she have any abnormal physical signs during an arrhythmia?
(c) Does she need treatment for this arrhythmia?

80

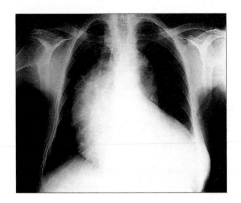

◀ 171

This 86-year-old woman had rheumatic fever as a child and is known to have valvular disease.

(a) How would you report this X-ray?

(b) Which chambers of the heart are particularly enlarged?

(c) Do these enlarged chambers confer any advantage to the patient?

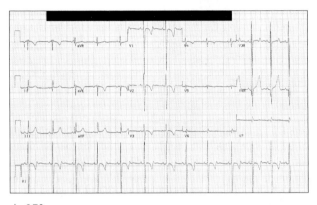

▲ 172

This patient was referred for an ECG because of palpitation; the referring doctor also mentioned a loud P2.

(a) How would you report the ECG?

(b) Why is P2 loud?

(c) What measure would you like to take to help assess the ECG?

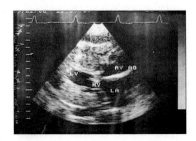

◀ 173

This 44-year-old man was found to have a heart murmur which was maximal in the aortic area.

(a) What abnormalities are present?

(b) What is the likely diagnosis?

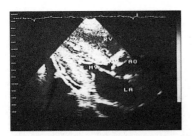

This 72-year-old man presents with high
venous pressure and a gallop rhythm.
(a) What view is displayed?
(b) Name four abnormalities.
(c) Why might the myocardium appear so
    echogenic?

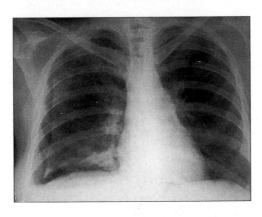

◀ 175
This 27-year-old drug addict
presented with a fever,
cough, and sputum
expectoration. She also had
withdrawal symptoms.
(a) How would you report
    the X-ray?
(b) Why does she have this
    abnormal X-ray?
(c) If the presenting con-
    dition recurs after treat-
    ment, what diagnosis
    would you consider?

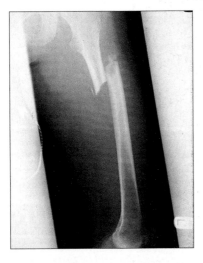

◀ 176
This X-ray was taken from a 65-year-old
man who fell from a high stepladder. He
was not found for some hours but when
he presented in Accident and Emergency
was in pain and was short of breath.
Physical examination of the cardiovascular
system was unremarkable apart from a
pulse rate of 110/minute. He had a
petechial skin rash.
(a) What does the X-ray show?
(b) Why might he have a skin rash?
(c) What investigation result would you
    like to know?
(d) Does this condition have a good
    prognosis?

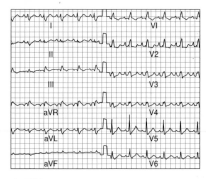

▲ 177

This 52-year-old woman presented with a history of palpitation. During the palpitations she becomes dizzy and has been reported to become very blue. She does not lose consciousness. Physical examination is normal and there is no clinical evidence of any chamber hypertrophy.

(a) What does the ECG show?

(b) Can you suggest why she might become dizzy with the arrhythmia?

(c) Why might she become cyanosed?

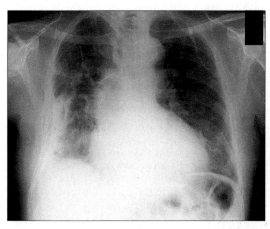

▲ 178

This X-ray is from a 68-year-old man who presented with atrial fibrillation and heart failure. Physical examination revealed him to have a mixture of aortic valve and mitral valve disease. He was extremely short of breath but responded to treatment.

(a) What are the abnormalities in the chest X-ray?

(b) How would you account for the abnormalities in the X-ray?

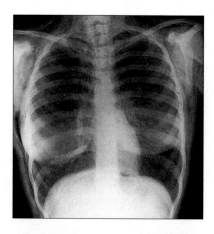

◀ 179

This 37-year-old woman was brought into the accident and emergency department extremely short of breath. She had a past history of asthma. Her additional complaint was that of swelling of the chest and neck.

(a) What are the abnormalities on the X-ray?
(b) Do the abnormalities need any particular treatment?
(c) Is this an unusual occurrence in asthma?

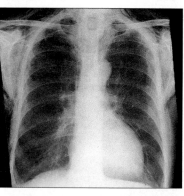

◀ 180

You are called to see this asthmatic patient. Some very abnormal heart sounds have been heard. The patient had a tachycardia but a normal blood pressure and was already responding to the treatment.

(a) What does the X-ray show?
(b) What might the explanation for the abnormal heart sounds be?
(c) Is there any specific action to be taken?

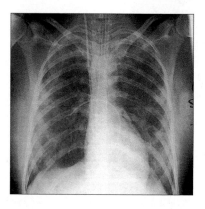

◀ 181

This 55-year-old woman was being treated for adult respiratory distress syndrome (ARDS) secondary to a septicemia. She is being ventilated and has reasonable blood gases at an FiO_2 of 0.40 (inspired O_2 concentration of 40%).

(a) She has an endotracheal tube *in situ*. There are two intravascular catheters. Where are they sited?
(b) What pressures can be measured via the two intravascular catheters?
(c) Why is it necessary to have these two catheters in place?

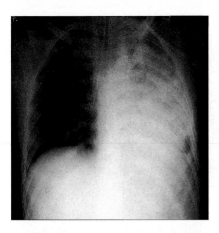

◀ 182

This 56-year-old man is brought to the intensive care unit (ICU) following a cardiac arrest. He had been intubated and was being ventilated. His BP was not satisfactory and he had a tachycardia of 120/minute.

(a) What does the X-ray show?
(b) What action needs to be taken?
(c) What physical sign is likely to be obvious when the patient first comes to the ICU?

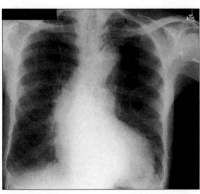

◀ 183

This 75-year-old man presents with increasing shortness of breath. He has been known to have a heart murmur for some time.

(a) What are the main abnormalities in the X-ray?
(b) What is the likeliest valvular abnormality?

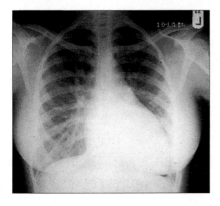

◀ 184

This 45-year-old woman presented with increasing shortness of breath. She had been known to have a murmur for many years.

(a) What are the main abnormalities?
(b) Which chamber of the heart bears the main load of this abnormality?
(c) What pathognomonic sign, which can be elicited from the end of the bed, may occur in this condition?

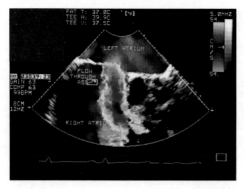

▲ 185

This woman, in her first pregnancy, was found to have a heart murmur at her first antenatal clinic appointment. She was totally asymptomatic. Her transesophageal echocardiogram demonstrates the atria, which are labeled.

(a) What is the physical basis of Doppler cardiography?

(b) What is the abnormality that has been demonstrated?

(c) What physical signs is she likely to have and what is the mechanism of them?

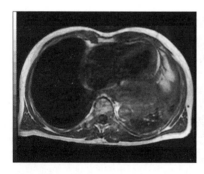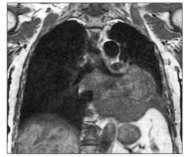

▲ 186

This nuclear magnetic resonance (NMR) image was obtained from a patient presenting with shortness of breath, weight loss, and a hoarse voice. Both the axial and coronal images are T_1 weighted.

(a) What is the main abnormality?

(b) Why might he have a hoarse voice?

(c) What is the likely etiology?

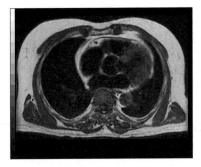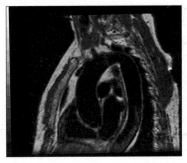

▲ 187

These NMR sagittal and oblique images are T_1 weighted. They were obtained from a young male who was referred for assessment with a BP of 155/110/110 mmHg in the right arm. A murmur had been heard in the outflow tract of the left ventricle and the referring clinician thought there might be some femoral delay.

(a) What diagnosis is the referring clinician suspicious of?

(b) How would you report the NMR images?

(c) The syndrome the referring clinician was considering has another component which would not be covered by this NMR scan. What is the other component?

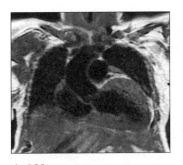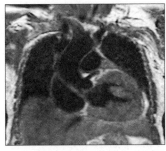

▲ 188

These NMR images were obtained from a 56-year-old man who was referred because of a mediastinal mass on the chest PA. These are coronal T_1-weighted images.

(a) What is the likeliest explanation for the mediastinal mass found on the chest PA?

(b) Are there any other abnormalities and how might you account for them?

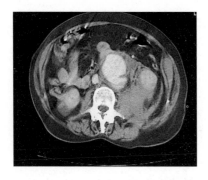

189

This CT scan of the abdomen was taken in a 75-year-old woman who presented acutely unwell with a sudden onset of faintness, sweating, and backache. Her BP on arrival was 70/50 mmHg; she had a tachycardia of 120/minute and looked pale.

(a) What is the main abnormality in the CT scan?
(b) What might be the correct management?
(c) What physical sign might have alerted the Accident and Emergency staff to her diagnosis?

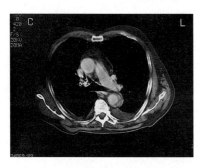

190

This 55-year-old man presented with chest pain which was thought to be cardiac in origin. His ECG was normal. His BP was 170/120/120 mmHg.

(a) What does the CT scan show?
(b) What is the likely diagnosis?
(c) What is the correct treatment?

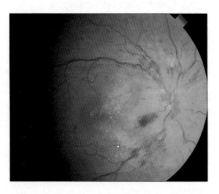

191

This picture of an optic disk was taken from a 43-year-old man who presented with palpitations and dizziness. He was also complaining of headaches.

(a) What do the optic fundi show?
(b) What term would you use to describe his condition?
(c) How would you treat this man's condition?

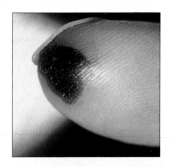

This 42-year-old man presented to outpatients with this uncomfortable lesion on his finger. There was no history of trauma.
(a) What is the likeliest cause of this lesion?
(b) What are the two most important investigations to perform?

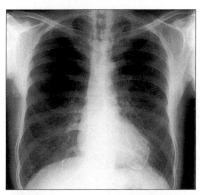

◀ 193

This 55-year-old man developed a chest infection which responded to anti-biotics. The primary care practitioner sent him for an X-ray.
(a) What does the X-ray show?
(b) What is the likeliest explanation of the abnormality?
(c) What treatment is indicated?

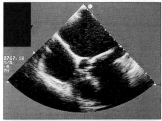

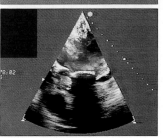

◀ 194

This transesophageal echocardiogram (TEE) was taken on a patient who had a mitral valve replacement with a prosthetic valve some 4 years previously. She started developing increasing heart failure 3 months before admission. A murmur was now audible in the mitral area. The top picture shows the ana-tomic structures and the lower the Doppler flows.
(a) What is the particular advantage of TEE over the more usual transthoracic echocardiography?
(b) What is the disadvantage of TEE over transthoracic echocardiography?
(c) What does this TEE show?
(d) What might be necessary for the patient?

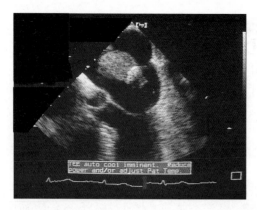

◀ 195

This TEE was taken from a patient who presented with splinter hemorrhages, low-grade fever and weight loss.

(a) What is the main abnormality in the TEE?

(b) What is the explanation for the abnormality?

(c) What should be done to treat the patient?

(d) Are there any other measures that should be taken?

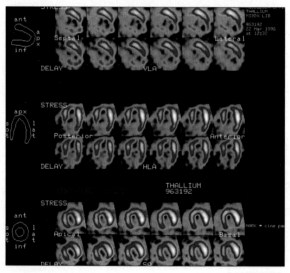

▲ 196

This 55-year-old man had noninsulin-dependent diabetes. Some years ago he suffered a myocardial infarction. He re-presented with angina which did not respond to medical treatment. His resting ECG was abnormal and showed an old inferior myocardial infarction and widespread ST-segment T-wave abnormalities in the anterior leads.

(a) Why might an exercise-thallium test have been performed rather than a standard exercise-stress test on a treadmill.

(b) What is the main abnormality?

(c) In the report mention was made of myocardial hibernation. What does this mean?

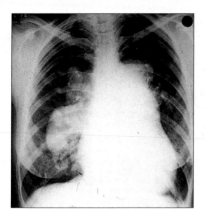

◀ 197

This 60-year-old woman complaining of progressively worsening shortness of breath had a heart murmur since the age of 24, when she was pregnant. She was not anemic, nor in heart failure, but had a tinge of cyanosis.

(a) Name four abnormalities here.
(b) What lesion might account for them?
(c) What options are available?

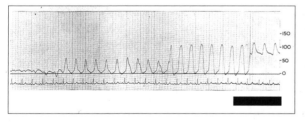

▲ 198

This 13-year-old patient had been cyanosed for at least 5 years. Pressure is measured in mmHg and the scale is shown. The recording is from the pulmonary artery to the right ventricle; it also shows the brachial artery pressure.

(a) Identify four abnormalities.
(b) Why is the patient cyanosed?
(c) What measures might the child take to improve oxygenation intermittently?
(d) What treatment might now be offered the patient for this condition?

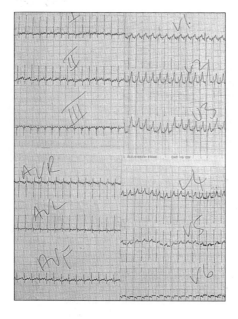

◀ 199

This 60-year-old man reported to the accident and emergency department with breathlessness and mild left-sided chest discomfort.

(a) How would you interpret the ECG?

(b) What action might you take?

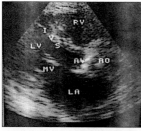

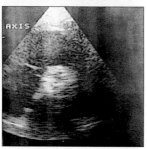

◀ 200

This woman presented with angina and was found to have a systolic murmur.

(a) What does the short-axis view of the aortic valve show?

(b) What does the long-axis view show?

(c) What is the likely explanation of her problems?

(d) Can any more information be gained about the severity of the condition by noninvasive means? Name three such means.

1   (a) Saphenous vein bypass graft. The internal mammary artery is increasingly being used as an alternative. It may give better symptom relief for a longer period of time although the operation itself is technically more difficult.
(b) The mortality rate should be between 1 and 3%. It is approximately twice as high in women.
(c) Approximately 50% of patients have angina again after 5 years which progressively rises to about 80% after 10 years; these figures are better if the internal mammary graft has been used.

2   (a) Complete AV block (third-degree AV block) with a high ventricular focus; this is consistent with a congenital etiology.
(b) The H deflection represents depolarization of the bundle of His and the V deflection the depolarization of the ventricles.
(c) The H–V interval can be useful in helping to predict the progression from first- or second-degree AV block to complete heart block; it can also be useful to someone who is having symptoms of syncope but whose electrocardiogram (ECG) is unhelpful.

3   (a) The intimal tear of an aortic dissection occurring just above the aortic valve.
(b) The dissection can track down towards, and then along, a coronary artery. This may cause myocardial ischemia or infarction, and ventricular fibrillation.
(c) Marfan's syndrome and systemic hypertension predispose to aortic dissection.

4   (a) High pulmonary artery wedge pressure (PAWP) and a diastolic pressure difference across the mitral valve. There is also a slow Y descent. This patient has severe mitral stenosis.
(b) Systemic embolization is a significant risk; the fact that the patient is in sinus rhythm does not remove the likelihood of embolization. Atrial fibrillation can be a very serious problem for a patient with this degree of mitral stenosis. Pulmonary edema may then develop and can sometimes result in death.
(c) The pulmonary artery pressure will be elevated; the extent of this elevation will depend on the pulmonary vascular resistance. It will be at least 35/20 mmHg but may be as high as 85/55 mmHg.

5   (a) The right coronary artery.
(b) It runs in the atrioventricular (AV) groove around to the back of the heart where, in about 80% of individuals, it gives off the branch to the AV node and the posterior descending coronary artery.
(c) The main branches are the conus artery, the right ventricular or acute marginal branch, the AV node branch, the posterior descending artery (in about 80% of individuals), and posterior ventricular branches.

ANSWERS

6   (a) A short PR interval; delta waves; repolarization abnormalities (abnormal ST segments and T waves); Q waves in the inferior leads.

b) Although he has the Wolff–Parkinson–White syndrome, the diagnosis of myocardial infarction will need to be excluded by other means such as enzymes. He actually had dyspepsia.

(c) A reciprocating atrial tachycardia; the impulses pass anterogradely down through the AV node and retrogradely back up the accessory bundle. These arrhythmias are usually benign and of nuisance value only. In a small group of patients who develop atrial fibrillation this is of more serious significance. It may be associated with the development of ventricular fibrillation and then sudden death. This group of patients need further electrophysiological investigations and may require ablation of the accessory bundle or long-term antiarrhythmic drug therapy.

7   (a) An enlarged heart; a large, smooth mediastinal mass; calcification within the mediastinal mass; opacification of the right upper zone of the lung.

(b) The mass is an aneurysm in the ascending aorta and also involving the arch; it is causing pressure on the esophagus and on the right upper-lobe bronchus. It has also caused widening of the aortic root thus causing aortic regurgitation.

(c) Syphilis.

8   (a) His AV block is intermittent; the pacemaker is on demand and his own complexes will therefore suppress any pacemaker impulses.

(b) A very fast pacing rate and a failure to capture (the third and fourth pacing artefacts do not capture the ventricle).

(c) The pacemaker needs to be changed.

9   (a) Eruptive xanthomata.

(b) On the buttocks.

(c) She probably has pancreatitis and resulting high lipid levels.

10   (a) Marked right-axis deviation; very large P waves suggesting right atrial enlargement; right bundle branch block; long PR interval.

(b) The palpitation is due to atrial tachyarrhythmias. Her atrial transport is very important to maintain right ventricular output; without it she becomes very unwell.

(c) With a high right atrial pressure due to her Ebstein's anomaly, she will shunt right to left through a patent foramen ovale or an atrial-septal defect . The anomaly is characterized by atrialization of part of the right ventricle; the remaining right ventricle may itself be abnormal. A large part of the output from the right side of the heart is therefore dependent on the right atrial contraction.

11 (a) There is free blood in the mediastinum and around the descending aorta. There is blood in the pleural space bilaterally but more on the left. The endotracheal tube lies with its tip in the right main bronchus.

(b) The most common vessel to be injured is the aorta. The most frequent problem is rupture just distal to the origin of the left subclavian artery; it can also rupture just proximal to the origin of the brachiocephalic artery. Occasionally there is avulsion of the vena cava.

(c) The definitive investigation would be an angiogram and this should be performed in a cardiothoracic center.

12 (a) She has differential cyanosis; her left hand and both legs are cyanosed while her right hand is normal. The reversed shunt of a patent ductus usually allows desaturated blood to enter the aorta just proximal to the origin of the left subclavian artery; it can sometimes enter just distal in which case the left arm will be a normal color.

(b) Polycythemia with its adverse effect on viscosity leading to thrombotic problems; hyperuricemia; paradoxical emboli; right heart failure; cerebral emboli.

(c) Once the shunt has reversed there is no place for closure of the duct. Certain drugs have been tried to attempt to reduce the pulmonary vascular resistance; they do not usually have a sustained effect although occasionally they can be dramatic in an individual. The only other treatment possibility is that of heart and lung transplantation.

13 (a) An atrial tachycardia with a 2:1 AV block, widespread ST-segment and T-wave abnormalities together with U waves.

(b) A serum potassium, which was 2.3 mmol/l.

(c) An infusion of 60 mmol potassium in 500 cc saline corrected the arrhythmia and improved the blood pressure.

14 (a) J waves; a bradycardia; shiver waves; a long QT interval; idioventricular rhythm.

(b) A rectal temperature, which was 32°C.

(c) Very gentle and slow rewarming, intravenous fluids and treatment of any precipitating factor such as a pneumonia, myocardial infarct, hypothyroidism.

(d) Arrhythmias; hypovolemia; pancreatitis; hypokalemia.

15 (a) There is a gradient within the cavity of the left ventricle. This is approximately 75 mmHg.

(b) The patient has either a hypertrophic obstructive cardiomyopathy, or subvalve aortic stenosis.

(c) At the bedside, the signs of an obstructive cardiomyopathy differ from those of subaortic stenosis. The echocardiogram may easily distinguish between them.

16   (a) Sinus rhythm with a normal PR interval; normal QRS axis; raised ST segments in leads I, V2–V6, this is maximal in V3–V5 and is associated with a high take off.

(b) Yes. It is a normal variant. It is found in males in all races and is becoming more recognized with the increased use of ECGs. It is extremely rare in women.

(c) Exercise will bring the ST segment down to the isoelectric line. Alternatively a small dose of intravenous atropine can be used which will produce the same effect. It is important, of course, to be certain that the ST-segment abnormality does not represent some more sinister pathology before embarking on these measures.

17   (a) Sinus tachycardia; QRS axis +80; slight right-bundle intraventricular conduction defect; T-wave inversion in V1–V3; T-wave inversion in III; an S1, Q3, T3 pattern.

(b) Although myocardial infarction is a possibility, the ECG is very right-sided and is more in keeping with a major pulmonary embolus.

(c) His venous pressure is already slightly high; nevertheless, he needs more filling in order to 'drive' his right ventricle. In addition, he needs treatment for the embolus; the choice of drug lies between heparin, streptokinase, or another thrombolytic agent. Most patients do very well with suitable doses of heparin. He will need pulmonary angiography and the catheter can be used to break up the embolism; the heparin or a thrombolytic agent can then be perfused directly into the pulmonary artery. Surgery has a very small role; it can be used if the patient fails to respond to medical treatment.

(d) Drugs that cause venous dilatation must be avoided; thus the opiates are contra-indicated. Chest discomfort is best dealt with by drugs such as aspirin, acetaminophen, or dihydrocodeine.

18   (a) The P wave and QRS morphology in lead I and a VR should alert you to the fact that the limb leads have been accidentally reversed. There is rather poor R wave progression across the chest leads, but this is not typical of dextrocardia.

(b) The ECG should be re-recorded with the limb leads correctly attached.

19   (a) The M-mode echocardiogram shows a wide amplitude of movement of the mitral valve. There is a prolapse or posterior displacement of the leaflet(s) in systole; this movement can vary both in amplitude and duration in the same patient at different times.

(b) Mitral valve prolapse. It is important to exclude the possibility of an underlying cardiomyopathy; the echocardiogram is a useful investigation for this condition. The prolapse is caused by myxomatous degeneration of the mitral valve and can be associated with chest pain and arrhythmias; historically it is therefore very important to exclude the possibility of myocardial ischemia. The murmur can vary markedly with different postures and may be inaudible at times; postures that increase LV wall tension will increase the intensity of the murmur.

(c) On the basis that the condition has been shown to be an isolated mitral valve abnormality due to myxomatous degeneration, the condition is almost always benign. Antibiotic cover needs to be given for potentially septic procedures.

20 (a) Scleroderma. The history in conjunction with the puckering around her mouth and the telangiectatic spots on her nose and cheek make this diagnosis very likely.
(b) Difficulty in swallowing.
(c) The most likely cause of her shortness of breath is associated pulmonary fibrosis. This can affect the heart; sometimes pulmonary hypertension can develop without much lung involvement. The heart can also be involved by a vasculitis which may produce fibrotic changes in the myocardium; pericarditis is also fairly common. The disease virtually never affects the heart valves.

21 (a) There is widespread ST-segment elevation with concavity upwards without any reciprocal changes.
(b) Pericarditis or peri-myocarditis is the most likely diagnosis. A myocardial infarction is unlikely because of the absence of any pathological Q waves and no reciprocal ST-segment depression.
(c) To avoid strenuous exertion for a period of 2 months; although the diagnosis is probably a pericarditis, there is also inflammation of the myocardium. Sudden death has been recorded in young people who have returned to energetic activities too soon.

22 (a) A thickened anterior leaflet which closes very slowly producing a reduced E-F slope; the posterior leaflet is not well seen but is probably not moving very much; the mitral valve ring is also very thickened.
(b) Mitral valve stenosis due to rheumatic heart disease. It is very difficult to judge the severity from the M-mode echocardiogram. The E–F slope and the relative slopes of the anterior and posterior leaflets have been used but do not give a very accurate estimate. The echocardiogram gives structural information and any attempt to gain hemodynamic data from it is fraught with difficulty. Echo/Doppler gives additional information about flow.
(c) One line corresponds to the opening snap and the other to the mitral valve closure, which may be loud. The latter occurs because the valve is snapped shut by the very rapidly rising left ventricular (LV) pressure which overcomes the elevated left atrial (LA) pressure. The opening snap occurs when the LV diastolic pressure falls below the elevated LA pressure.

23 (a) 96–99% saturation.
(b) Left upper pulmonary vein. IVC-> RA-> LA-> PV; the passage through the atrial septum is either through a patent foramen ovale or an atrial-septal defect.
(c) It will be the same as the LA pressure which in the normal person is 8–12 mmHg.

24   (a) There is a pressure difference within the aorta; the catheter is withdrawn from the LV (with a low diastolic pressure) into the aorta; there is no difference in the systolic pressure between LV and aorta (i.e. there is no aortic valve stenosis). However, on withdrawing a little further into the aorta there is a pressure drop of about 70 mmHg.

(b) This could occur in a supravalvar aortic stenosis or in a coarctation of the aorta.

25   (a) Bizarre QRS complexes. Bradycardia which is probably idioventricular. Long QT interval.

(b) A drug overdose containing the tricyclics is a likely possibility.

(c) She is highly likely to develop a *torsade de pointes*. This is a ventricular tachycardia with a changing QRS axis. It does not respond to conventional anti-arrhythmic therapy and isoprenaline may be necessary.

26   (a) The midline scar of the sternotomy and pronounced gynecomastia.

(b) Spironolactone and digoxin.

(c) The breasts can become painful.

27   (a) She has an extra digit on her left hand together with some hypoplasia of the fifth finger.

(b) Polydactyly can be associated with congenital heart disease.

(c) Yes. The two best known conditions in which polydactyly occurs in association with congenital heart disease are Laurence–Moon–Biedl syndrome and Ellis–van Creveld syndrome. The former is inherited as a recessive and is associated with obesity, mental retardation, renal problems and retinitis pigmentosa. The latter is inherited as a recessive and is characterized by dwarfism.

28   (a) The xanthelasma are composed of lipid.

(b) She has an obvious arcus. In a young woman the presence of an arcus is highly suggestive of an underlying lipoprotein abnormality.

(c) On the basis that she has been shown to have significant hypercholesterolemia it is important to do the following: (i) check that she does not have any other risk factors for coronary artery disease (if she does then these need treatment or advice); (ii) embark on the appropriate treatment for her lipid abnormality (in the first instance this will be dietary but she will almost certainly need to have drug treatment as well); (iii) her first-degree relatives must also be checked for lipid abnormalities and any other risk factors.

29 (a) Le main d'accoucheur is produced by inducing latent tetany by occluding the arterial supply to the forearm (Trousseau's sign).
(b) The QT interval will be prolonged; this interval will need to be corrected for heart rate (QTc).
(c) Ventricular arrhythmias occur; one of the described arrhythmias is the *torsade de pointes* which may be mistaken for a conventional ventricular tachyarrhythmia; it is important to recognize it since its treatment differs markedly from that of the conventional ventricular tachyarrhythmia.

30 (a) There is considerable widening of the mediastinum; the appearances are more in keeping with enlargement of mediastinal glands than with a vascular cause. The heart is also a little enlarged but the lung fields are clear.
(b) She has the classic signs of tamponade: a paradoxical pulse, an inspiratory rise in the venous pressure, and a tachycardia. Treatment by pericardiocentesis is urgently required to relieve the tamponade.
(c) With the given story and investigations a lymphoma is the most likely etiology. Tuberculosis must not be overlooked as a possibility.
(d) The paradox is that, as the patient inspires, the heart rate increases but the pulse rate apparently reduces or disappears.

31 (a) He has one of the mucopolysaccharidoses. He has type II (McCusick's classification) or Hunter's disease; this is inherited on a sex-linked recessive basis.
(b) Hepatosplenomegaly, dorsolumbar kyphosis, progressive joint stiffness, swelling, and contractures.
(c) There is deposition of the glycoprotein in both the myocardium and in the valves, particularly the mitral valve.

32 (a) They are xanthelasma.
(b) Xanthelasma in this age group are often not associated with any lipid abnormality or with any vascular disease.
(c) An arcus at this age is of no significance. The prevalence of an arcus rises with age; in women over the age of 50 an arcus is just as likely to be associated with normal or low levels of lipids as with high levels of lipids. There is no association with vascular disease.

33 (a) The word which best describes it is the French word *accrochage*, meaning hitching up to or coupling. This is a form of AV dissociation where the P wave moves in and out of the QRS complex and normal AV conduction takes place for a few beats.
(b) This is a benign arrhythmia and the patient can be reassured.

ANSWERS

34 (a) The ECG shows sinus rhythm with a normal PR interval. The mean QRS axis is towards the right and is $+110^0$. There is poor R-wave progression across the chest leads. There is an extremely short QT and QTc interval with virtual obliteration of any ST segment. There is also generalized flattening of the T waves. The ECG is consistent with hypercalcemia; the QRS axis raises the possibility of some right ventricle (RV) hypertrophy.

(b) The chest condition could be a carcinoma or, more likely, sarcoid giving rise to hypercalcemia. If there were extensive lung involvement then RV hypertrophy might be expected to develop.

35 (a) She has tendon xanthoma.

(b) Severe hypercholesterolemia can present with an arthropathy which will affect the ankle joints particularly, but can also involve other joints. Xanthoma are usually present in the Achilles tendon.

(c) She has the heterozygous form of familial hypercholesterolemia (FH). She therefore has only half the number of effective low-density lipoprotein (LDL) receptors on her cell membrane. As a result, the intracellular level of cholesterol is low, thus stimulating the further production of cholesterol; these factors produce the high blood levels and the tissue deposition.

36, 37

(a) Meningococcal septicemia. This condition can be rapidly fatal. It would be useful to know whether there were any other cases of meningococcal infections around. Having taken throat swabs and blood for culture, clotting screen, white count, and for the antigen, intravenous antibiotic treatment should be started immediately. The drug of choice is intravenous penicillin in a dose of 4 mega units every 6 hours.

(b) The low blood pressure is an ominous sign. It is related to the endotoxemia. Although the occasional patient may develop adrenal hemorrhage and the Waterhouse–Friderichsen syndrome, the vast majority have a normal adrenal response to stress. The meningococcus endotoxin is a most potent endotoxin in producing damage to cutaneous blood vessels. The measures to control hypotension include expansion of the plasma volume and the use of inotropes. The central venous and left atrial pressures may need to be kept quite high since impaired cardiac function may be a consequence of the endotoxemia.

(c) It is important to trace contacts of the patient and to treat them or vaccinate them as appropriate.

38 (a) Sinus rhythm with a normal PR interval; normal QRS axis; widespread upwardly concave ST-segment elevation without any reciprocal ST-segment depression. These changes are very suggestive of pericarditis.

(b) There are quite deep Q waves in III and a VF- together with a dominant R-wave in V1; this raises the possibility of an inferior infarct. However, the Q waves are probably within normal limits and the dominant R wave relates to the rotation of the heart in the horizontal plane.

(c) Although called acute benign pericarditis it can proceed to tamponade and death. This is an unusual complication but nevertheless needs to be watched for.

39 (a) There is a single ventricle. In the view through the atrioventricular valves both the mitral and tricuspid valves are seen but there is no interposed IV (interventricular) septum.

(b) The single ventricle functions as a common mixing chamber for both saturated and desaturated blood.

(c) The condition can be associated with pulmonary stenosis or atresia. Alternatively, it may be associated with asplenia.

40 (a) The ECG shows a sinus tachycardia with a normal PR interval. There are pathologic Q waves with ST-segment elevation in the inferior and lateral leads. There is reciprocal ST-segment depression in I and aVL.

(b) The cause of the hypotension must first be elucidated. Extensive myocardial necrosis is only one of the possibilities. Another important possibility to diagnose is that of a low left ventricular filling pressure; this may result from venodilatation caused by opiates or diuresis caused by strong diuretics such as furosemide. Both of the latter problems will respond to a fluid challenge. High venous pressure must not put one off this line of therapy. High venous pressure is probably caused by the RV infarct, in which case treatment will be determined according to the measurement of the left atrial filling pressure. Treatment may involve the use of inotropes, or vasodilators, or both.

(c) It is now thought that the reciprocal ST-segment depression reflects a large infarct. At one stage it was thought that it might represent coronary artery disease in another territory; this has now been largely disproved.

41 (a) The ECG shows a sinus tachycardia with a normal PR interval. There is an S1, Q3, T3 pattern. The QRST complexes are otherwise normal. This ECG is normal for someone who is pregnant. There is no evidence of acute right-heart strain.

(b) There is a 30% increase in the circulating volume and cardiac output; this starts early in pregnancy and reaches a plateau at the end of the first trimester. It remains elevated for the remainder of the pregnancy and does not decrease in the last trimester, as was once thought. There is also a reduction in the systemic resistance resulting in a lowered blood pressure.

(c) The circulating blood volume and cardiac output increase by a further 30%; this begins to fall over the first few hours but, particularly if the mother is breast-feeding, does not return to the pre-pregnancy levels for some weeks.

42   (a) There is a saccular aneurysm arising from the descending aorta. She has calcification in her trachea, bronchi, and aortic knuckle.
(b) This is likely to be atheroma.
(c) Unless there was demonstrable expansion of the aneurysm, no specific treatment has been shown to be of merit. If she were hypertensive, then this should be appropriately treated.

43   (a) A very dilated aortic root. There is a clearly seen flap extending from just above the aortic valve around the arch and down the descending aorta. This is the interface between the true and the false lumens. He has a dissection starting in the classic site just above the aortic valve and extending down the descending aorta and also up the carotid artery. This is a type-I dissection.
(b) The first measures are to stabilize the blood pressure and ensure the systolic pressure is in the region of 100 mmHg; in this man hypertension was not a problem. Beta-blockers are also used in order to reduce the shearing force of systole. After delineating the type of dissection and the site of the tear, the treatment of choice, in this instance, is surgical.
(c) Systemic hypertension, Marfan's syndrome, and pregnancy.

44   (a) The MRI of his brain shows an abnormal signal in the inferior part of the right cerebellar hemisphere which is compatible with a mature infarction.
(b) The clinician needs to be on the alert to the development of hydrocephalus.
(c) The MRI scan is the best investigation to demonstrate brain stem and cerebellar problems.

45   (a) The end-diastolic pressure in the left ventricle is elevated; the left atrial pressure is elevated; there is a large V wave or systolic wave in the LA tracing.
(b) The elevated end-diastolic pressure is indicative of heart failure. The large systolic wave, which is much larger than the A wave, reflects mitral regurgitation. It is difficult, with the limited history and other information given, to be certain of the diagnosis. The patient had a dilated cardiomyopathy and then developed quite severe mitral regurgitation. The patient subsequently had a successful mitral valve replacement and his symptoms improved considerably.
(c) A ruptured chorda tendinea. The patient also had a mitral valve that had myxomatous degeneration. Other causes to consider are infective endocarditis, papillary muscle dysfunction, and a dilated valve ring associated with the cardiomyopathy.

46 (a) The ECG shows a regular tachycardia which is probably a sinus tachycardia. There is marked ST-segment elevation in I, II, III, and aVF with ST-segment depression in V2. The QRS axis is normal for this age and there is no evidence of any chamber hypertrophy.

(b) A myocarditis is the most likely explanation. An anomalous coronary artery originating from the pulmonary trunk is worth considering but does not usually present in this manner. The child was confirmed to have a coxsackie B myocarditis.

(c) Heart failure in this age group can be caused by a myocarditis which may be due to the coxsackie virus or echovirus. Other causes include congenital heart disease and aortic regurgitation. Congenital complete-heart block or supraventricular tachycardia may also cause heart failure, as may arteriovenous shunts. Endocardial fibroelastosis usually presents a little later but can present at this early age. The majority of infants who develop heart failure within the first week of life will do so as a result of critical obstruction of systemic arterial flow, such as aortic atresia or coarctation.

47 (a) Aortic valve stenosis; supravalve aortic stenosis; subvalve aortic stenosis; coarctation of the aorta. An obstructive cardiomyopathy would produce a pressure difference between the LV cavity and the outflow tract but the femoral pulse tracing would be expected to be more 'jerky' in character than the one displayed.

(b) The pressure difference is about 75 mmHg, which is severe.

(c) Lower. The normal aorta relaxes to accommodate the volume of blood expressed from the ventricle during systole. During systole the aorta recoils, thus helping the propulsion of blood distally; this results in the apparent paradox of the femoral artery pressure actually being slightly higher than the aortic pressure.

48 (a) On the PA (posteroanterior) film the right hilum is abnormal. There is a smooth rounded mass at the right hilum which appears to have blood vessels joining it. There may be similar but smaller lesions at the left hilum. On a lateral the rounded mass can be seen at the hilum; again, vessels appear to be joining it. The heart is slightly enlarged. The most likely explanation is that these lesions are vascular and are pulmonary arteriovenous fistulae.

(b) Cardiac catheterization and angiography. A pulmonary angiogram would display the lesion.

(c) The manifestations and complications depend on the size and number of the atrioventricular (AV) malformations. If large, they can present in infancy with cyanosis and heart failure. They can be multiple and part of the Rendu–Osler–Weber syndrome. The other complications are those associated with cyanosis.

ANSWERS

49 (a) This is an atrial myxoma. It usually arises from, and is attached to, the interatrial septum. As it grows it develops a stalk. It can interfere with the function of the mitral valve. It can, as in this woman, be responsible for cerebral emboli.

(b) It can mimic mitral valve disease. It can produce intermittent obstruction of the mitral and other valves. It can sometimes present as a low-grade fever and mimic infective endocarditis. It can present as an embolic problem.

(c) Two-dimensional (2-D) echocardiography is the best investigation. Angiography is now rarely required.

50 (a) Aortic valve.

(b) The valve is likely to have caused obstruction to outflow, as well as remaining as a relatively fixed orifice which could not close in diastole. The murmurs were mid-systolic of a crescendo–decrescendo type and an immediate diastolic murmur.

(c) The valve is calcified and this was apparent over the vertebrae on the PA film. The ascending aorta was prominent, reflecting the post-stenotic dilatation. The heart was not enlarged since stenosis was the dominant lesion and hypertrophy does not usually produce enlargement of the cardiac silhouette.

51 (a) The specificity of an exercise-stress test on a treadmill is not very good in women. An alternative explanation might be that she has an abnormal resting ECG.

(b) The images obtained after stress and after a delay are identical. The test is quite normal.

(c) The thallium-stress test result can be used as reassurance. Alternatively, it will provoke the search for alternative explanations for her chest discomfort.

52 (a) There is sinus tachycardia. There are changes of an acute anterior myocardial infarction and also an acute inferior infarction.

(b) This man has sustained a very large myocardial infarction. Nevertheless, there is likely to be quite a lot of salvageable myocardium which is currently 'stunned'. The first measure to be established is whether his filling pressures on the left side are adequate; a Swan–Ganz catheter needs to be inserted and his filling optimized. Consideration can then be given to raising his blood pressure with an inotrope. The other measure that should be considered, if medical treatment does not help, is use of the balloon support system.

(c) He is at very high risk of dying within the first year of his infarct. Medical measures that may reduce this risk include the use of angiotensin-converting enzyme (ACE) inhibitors, lowering of blood cholesterol with statins, and the use of aspirin. There is no good evidence that surgery or angioplasty has a part to play in prolonging his life unless he were to become symptomatic.

53   (a) Sinoatrial node branch; right ventricular branch (also called acute marginal); branch to AV node; posterior LV branch; posterior descending branch.

(b) The right coronary artery has some disease in it; the walls are a little irregular but there are no critical stenoses. There is cross-filling to the anterior descending territory; this is consistent with disease in this artery. Unfortunately the collaterals do not prevent angina but may reduce the likelihood of a large myocardial infarct in that territory.

(c) The mortality rate will vary with the population under study. If a high proportion of patients studied have mild disease or normal arteries, then the mortality will be very low. In the UK the mortality is about 2 in 1000 studies.

54   (a) The left-hand part of both rhythm strips, which are continuous, show a rhythm which might be sinus tachycardia. It then degenerates rapidly into a ventricular tachycardia or even a ventricular flutter. This latter rhythm would not be associated with an output.

(b) Cardiopulmonary resuscitation should be commenced immediately. The patient may need defibrillation as the rhythm degenerates further. Whenever possible, the patient should be moved to an environment, such as the accident and emergency department, where he can be appropriately treated thereafter.

(c) This will depend on the underlying disease process and whether it can be corrected. In fact he had underlying ischemic heart disease and required bypass surgery. Thereafter, he had no further rhythm abnormalities.

55   (a) Total opacifictation of the left hemithorax; mediastinal shift towards the left; overexpansion of the right hemithorax.

(b) An obstruction to the left main bronchus due to the endotracheal tube being too far down the right main bronchus; the anesthetist had just pulled the tube back. Alternatively, there could be a mucous plug or foreign body obstructing the bronchus.

(c) Physiotherapy may be all that is required to unblock the bronchus and allow re-expansion. Endobronchial aspiration should also be performed. If these measures fail, bronchoscopy will be necessary.

56   (a) Enlarged heart; enlarged left atrium; enlarged right atrium; calcification in left atrial wall.

(b) The right atrial border is very prominent; this suggests the presence of tricuspid incompetence. The tricuspid incompetence could be on the basis of rheumatic involvement of the tricuspid valve or it could be secondary to right-heart failure due to high pulmonary artery pressures.

(c) The Starr–Edwards valve will produce an opening sound; the timing of this will be similar to that of the opening snap of mitral stenosis. The closing sound will occur with the first heart sound.

ANSWERS

57 (a) The most important difference is the upper mediastinum which has enlarged. The shape of the enlargement suggests a glandular basis.

(b) An enlarged left atrium can press on the esophagus and cause dysphagia.

(c) Histology is important to obtain. It is unlikely that either bronchoscopy or endoscopy will give this. A mediastinoscopy and biopsy is probably the most fruitful investigation.

58 (a) The X-ray shows a large heart. The pulmonary arteries are all large which suggests a left-to-right shunt.

(b) It was a continuous murmur of a patent ductus arteriosus. It was well heard in the pulmonary area but was also loud under the left clavicle.

(c) The definitive investigation would be cardiac-catheter study and angiography. The study would show a step-up in oxygen saturation at pulmonary artery level. The size of the left-to-right shunt can be calculated. In this instance there was a pulmonary/systemic flow ratio of 4:1. The aortogram demonstrated the duct in the classic site.

59 (a) It is difficult to comment on the heart size in a PA erect film. There is soft intra-alveolar shadowing in both lung fields. This is very suggestive of pulmonary edema. A pneumonic process is an alternative but the bilateral nature and the hilar flare suggest otherwise.

(b) On the basis that this is pulmonary edema, the next question is to determine whether it is related to heart failure or to other causes. The gallop rhythm and hemodynamic changes suggest that it is due to heart failure. An acute myocarditis is a possibility and the recent chest infection would be consistent with this; the ECG is against this diagnosis. A prolonged arrhythmia must be excluded, as must a metabolic problem causing the acidosis. A recent myocardial infarction can be easily excluded as a cause. Acute mitral regurgitation might cause a picture of severe pulmonary edema; however, there was no murmur.

(c) It is most unusual not to get some response to the measures described. The severe degree of acidosis and resistant heart failure must raise the possibility of thiamine deficiency. He had Shoshin beriberi and responded dramatically to thiamine.

60 (a) Long runs of ventricular tachycardia. Numerous ventricular premature beats. There are several fusion beats seen.

(b) No, but the appearance of fusion beats in the context of the very abnormal QRS complexes makes it 90–98% certain that this is ventricular in origin.

(c) No. Contrary to popular belief a ventricular tachycardia is often as well tolerated as a supraventricular tachycardia at equivalent rates. The main determinant of the presence of symptoms is likely to be the actual rate and the function of the heart, rather than the mechanism of the arrhythmia.

61   (a) Although it is an erect, portable film, the heart appears large. The mediastinum is very wide. There is some shadowing at the left base which may be fluid.

(b) A dissection of the aorta is a distinct possibility. Blood pressure in both arms and legs will need to be checked. The next investigation of choice will depend on the local facilities. A transthoracic echocardiogram, performed by a skilled person, might be able to demonstrate the dissection if it involves the aortic root. A transesophageal echocardiogram, if available, may well be the best investigation. A CT scan can be a useful investigation. An aortogram should only be done in a cardiothoracic center, but will give the necessary detailed information for the surgeon. If the index of suspicion is high, the patient should be transferred to a cardiothoracic center for an aortogram.

(c) His blood pressure needs to be brought down with intravenous nitroprusside infusion to a systolic of 100 mmHg. Beta-blocking drugs should be given to reduce the shearing stress of the aorta. Opiate analgesia should be given for the relief of discomfort, should it recur.

62   (a) Immunologic response from which no culture can be obtained.

(b) Septic focus from which cultures could be obtained.

(c) Septicemia with probable infective endocarditis.

63   (a) The waves are (i) the 'a' wave related to atrial contraction; (ii) the x descent related to atrial relaxation and the downward movement of the AV valves; (iii) the 'v' wave related to atrial filling; (iv) the y descent related to ventricular filling; (v) the 'c' wave related to the downward movement of the AV valves; (vi) the 'h' wave relates to the high diastolic pressure.

(b) There is a strikingly sharp y descent.

(c) Constrictive pericarditis. An alternative might be a tricuspid incompetence but one would expect a large systolic wave preceding the y descent.

64   (a) She has a normal sized heart. The shape of the left heart border suggests an enlarged left atrium and pulmonary artery. There is upper-lobe diversion indicative of a raised left atrial pressure.

(b) She has mitral stenosis and a high left atrial pressure.

(c) Atrial fibrillation; systemic embolization; pulmonary arterial hypertension; hemoptysis; pulmonary edema.

65   (a) The interventricular septum is very thick. The anterior leaflet of the mitral valve is fluttering.

(b) The fluttering of the anterior leaflet is caused by aortic regurgitation. He has the murmur of aortic regurgitation and an Austin Flint murmur.

(c) The regurgitant jet of blood through the leaking aortic valve impinges on the open anterior leaflet of the mitral valve causing it to flutter in a characteristic way.

66   (a) Although this looks like ventricular fibrillation it is often resistant to the therapy that one would normally use. It is a *torsade de pointes*. The serum potassium must be checked and corrected if necessary. DC (Direct Current) version may have a temporary effect. Drugs that prolong the QT interval should be avoided since they tend to make matters worse.

(b) It is worth trying the effect of treating the patient with a drug such as isoprenaline given intravenously. Overdrive pacing is another way of handling this problem; the pacemaker rate is set well above the inherent rhythm and it effectively suppresses the ectopic focus.

(c) Complete AV block. Drugs that prolong the QT interval such as quinidine, procainamide, amiodarone, phenothiazines, and insecticides. Hypokalemia or hypomagnesemia. Congenital QT prolongation.

67   (a) A systolic murmur in the phonocardiogram. In the echocardiogram there is a thick IV septum, systolic anterior movement (SAM) of the mitral valve and early closure of the aortic valve. There is also a reduced diastolic closure rate of the mitral valve.

(b) Hypertrophic obstructive cardiomyopathy.

(c) Treatment is necessary to try to reduce the progress of the hypertrophy and also to prevent arrhythmias. The former may be helped by calcium-channel blocking drugs, the latter by drugs such as amiodarone or beta-blockers. If the patient has angina then beta-blockers are of particular value.

68, 69

(a) Infective endocarditis. There are numerous vegetations on the mitral valve.

(b) 30% of patients with this condition still die. If the initial presentation is with a neurological picture such as a 'stroke' or confusional state, the risk of death is in excess of 50%. In the elderly the risk of death is about 50%. The longer the interval between the onset of symptoms and the diagnosis and initiation of good treatment, the worse the outcome.

(c) First consider the possibility of infective endocarditis, then examine the patient carefully for clinical evidence of the condition. The next step is to take two or three sets of blood cultures; the ideal time to take these is when the patient's temperature rises. There is little to be gained in taking more than three cultures. Examination of a specimen of fresh urine for red cells is also a useful investigation. Although an echocardiogram can confirm a diagnosis, a negative test does not exclude the possibility of infective endocarditis.

(d) Intravenous antibiotics. The particular antibiotic will depend on the clinical picture and the bacteriologic evidence. The adequacy of treatment must be checked with the aid of the microbiologists and the use of back-titration techniques. These test whether serial dilutions of the patient's serum will inhibit and kill the actual organism isolated. The duration and route of administration of the antibiotics will depend on this information.

70 (a) The ventricle is large and poorly moving. The mitral valve is opening only with atrial systole. The aortic root is not moving, which is consistent with a poor cardiac output. The aortic valve leaflets float together during systole; this also suggests a poor output.
(b) The patient has a dilated heart with very poor LV function.
(c) A postviral cardiomyopathy or alcohol excess are possibilities. Even in the absence of angina or other evidence of coronary artery disease, this picture could be caused by coronary artery disease. In most patients the specific etiology cannot be determined.

71 (a) There is significant ST-segment depression in the anterolateral and inferior leads. This is consistent with underlying exercise-induced ischemia.
(b) In a hospital population in the UK, the sensitivity for women is about 70% and the specificity about 55%; this is much less than for men. The reason is not fully understood.
(c) Yes. The systolic blood pressure should progressively rise with increasing severity of exercise. If it does not rise, the exercise test should be stopped because it indicates that the ventricle is seriously malfunctioning.

72 (a) A very loud first heart sound; a close opening snap; P2 is loud, a long diastolic murmur with presystolic accentuation.
(b) The very close opening snap (0.06 seconds) and the long murmur suggest that this is severe mitral stenosis. The loud P2 suggests that there is pulmonary hypertension.
(c) The cardiac output and circulating blood volume start to rise soon after the beginning of pregnancy and reach a peak by the end of the 10th week. They then remain constant and do not reduce. At the time of delivery the cardiac output increases by another 30%. The danger times for a woman with mitral stenosis are therefore near the beginning of pregnancy or very soon after delivery.

73 (a) An early systolic click; an early diastolic click; a short systolic murmur after the systolic click.
(b) The clicks are produced by prosthetic valves such as a Starr–Edwards valve. The aortic prosthetic valve will produce the systolic click and short systolic murmur. The mitral prosthetic valve will produce the diastolic click as the valve opens.
(c) These prosthetic valves may produce emboli and the patient has to be anticoagulated. They may produce hemolysis. Very occasionally the ball of the tilting mechanism may get stuck in a particular position. They are, of course, prone to get infected but no more so than a diseased valve, a homograft, or a heterograft replacement.

74   (a) High right ventricular pressure; slightly high right atrial pressure; step-up in oxygen saturation at ventricular level; step-down in oxygen saturation at left ventricular level; desaturated blood in aorta.

(b) Pulmonary stenosis and a ventricular septal defect; the Fallot situation.

(c) Polycythemia; gout; high viscosity; endocarditis; paradoxical emboli; syncope; arrhythmias may lead to death.

75   (a) There is a yellow discoloration in the skin folds and creases. These are xanthomata.

(b) He probably has a type-III or broad beta-band hyperlipoproteinemia. The acuteness of its onset suggests that this is probably associated with an acute illness, such as pancreatitis, rather than a genetically determined abnormality.

(c) Initially treat the underlying condition, such as pancreatitis. If this is a primary abnormality it will usually respond to the fibrate group of drugs.

76   (a) Aortic valve is thickened; left atrium is large; mitral valve is thickened and has reduced diastolic closure rate; IV septum and LV posterior wall are thickened.

(b) Aortic stenosis and mitral valve disease.

(c) The aortic valve disease may be severe in the light of the amount of LV hypertrophy. The mitral valve disease is difficult to assess; the large left atrium may be due to the rheumatic process rather than to severe regurgitation. The mitral stenosis is likely to be mild since the posterior leaflet is moving in the normal direction.

77   (a) Elevated left ventricular end-diastolic pressure (LVEDP); elevated PAWP; elevated pulmonary artery and right ventricular pressures.

(b) A myocardial problem.

(c) Idiopathic cardiomyopathy; alcoholic heart disease; coronary artery disease; post viral; drug-related, e.g. cobalt or duanorubicin.

78, 79

(a) There is coagulation necrosis present. This is characterized by the presence of the dead fibers which are hyaline and structureless. This appearance develops after about 8 hours of the event. Subsequent changes include the invasion of polymorphs, and after a few days the digestion of dead fibers by macrophages. The dead muscle is then replaced by fibrous tissue.

(b) Occlusion of a coronary artery causing myocardial infarction.

(c) The coagulation necrosis is evident at about 8 hours. There are a number of histochemical markers that have been used to try to determine much earlier changes. Although not entirely reliable, the use of nitroblue tetrazolium or triphenyl tetrazolium chloride can detect ischemic myocardium at 3 hours after the event.

80   (a) Pulmonary plethora and a slightly enlarged heart.

(b) The patent ductus arteriosus (PDA) puts a volume load in the left ventricle. Only when pulmonary vascular disease develops does the right ventricle have an additional load.

(c) Surgical management. The heart is already large because of the volume load and needs to be relieved of the high volume load.

81   (a) With the given history the most likely sequence is that of fat emboli leading to hypoxia; the analgesia made this worse, causing a hypoxic cardiac arrest. The other possibility might be related to the withdrawal effects from alcohol; a chest infection in these circumstances is not unusual and could produce hypoxia leading to cardiac arrest. Although there is no suggestion of a head injury, it obviously must be excluded.

(b) After fat emboli the two most difficult complications to deal with will be disseminated intravascular coagulation or adult respiratory distress syndrome (ARDS). The withdrawal effects from alcohol or other drugs can be very difficult to manage in a sick patient.

82   (a) The sensitivity and specificity are better. This particularly applies for women. It is very useful when the resting cardiogram is abnormal since a conventional exercise-stress test has to be interpreted with great caution. The exercise-thallium test allows a better correlation with the area of the myocardium that is ischemic.

(b) Entirely normal.

(c) The degree of radiation is equivalent to that of a barium enema. It is slightly more protracted for the patient. It is more expensive.

83   (a) There is a large mass within the left atrium which moves down towards the left ventricle on the lower frame. It is almost certainly a left atrial myxoma. It could be a different form of tumor. The valve looks quite normal.

(b) Embolic phenomena are very common. The diagnosis of a myxoma should be at least considered in every patient presenting with an embolism.

(c) Surgical removal.

(d) The tumor may recur. There may also be other members of the family with a myxoma.

ANSWERS

84 (a) The patient is in atrial fibrillation. There is an echogenic mass moving through the mitral valve in diastole and back into the left atrium in systole. The valve cusps themselves look normal and are not thickened. This could be an atrial myxoma or other cardiac tumor.

(b) Mitral regurgitation can occur because of the interference with the mitral valve function by the tumor. The movement of the tumor can produce an audible 'plop' which can be confused with an opening snap.

(c) The narrowed single beam makes the interpretation of anatomy difficult. It takes a well-trained technician to produce good and reliable results. There is a need to learn to recognize the pattern of the tracing in contradistinction to 2-D where the actual movements of structures are visualized.

85 (a) The patient has atrial flutter with a variable AV block. The heart rate is 120/minute. It is difficult to interpret the ST-segment and T-wave changes.

(b) One of the problems with atrial flutter is the sudden change in AV conduction allowing marked alteration in the heart rate; the heart tolerates poorly this sudden change in heart rate.

(c) The flutter waves will produce characteristic F waves in the venous pulse.

86 (a) Marked sinus arrhythmia; widespread ST-segment elevation without any reciprocal ST-segment depression or Q waves.

(b) Yes. A rise in inspiration suggests some cardiac compression.

(c) A paradoxical pulse; an inspiratory fall in the pulse pressure greater than 15 mmHg on inspiration. This would be of serious significance and indicate the need for pericardial aspiration.

87 (a) Left anterior fascicular block. Anticlockwise rotation.

(b) He ought to be monitored, but there is no indication to put in a cardiac pacemaker.

(c) Fibrosis of the conducting system. It is unlikely to be related to coronary artery disease although he may have coexisting disease. Fibrosis is part of the pathology of presbycardia or 'old person's heart'.

88 (a) The ECG is normal. Although there is quite a lot of voltage (R in V6 + S in V1 > 35 mm), this is normal for a slim, healthy young man.

(b) A normal ECG does not rule out the possibility of a cardiovascular problem. The test is very nonspecific and care has to be taken in ascribing either too much or too little importance to it.

112

89 (a) The high sampling rates from the two piezoelectric crystals make the continuous-wave Doppler an ideal technique for recording high flow velocities.

(b) Pulsed Doppler. In this mode there is only one piezoelectric crystal which alternates as a transmitter and a receiver. A burst of ultrasound is emitted by the transducer which then receives the signals from the depth of interest. The return signal is analyzed for Doppler shifts for a very brief time period; accordingly shifts in frequency can be determined very accurately at specific points along the beam. Its limitation is its relatively slow sampling rates for high-velocity flow.

(c) Yes. The flow is towards the transducer and therefore shown above the line. Normal flow through an aortic valve may be 1.0–1.5 m/second. In this instance the maximum flow is less than this; the aortic stenosis can be presumed to be minimal. Poor LV function may reduce the flow through a diseased aortic valve and therefore cause its severity to be underestimated.

90 (a) The waveform in systole is laminar and reflects flow through the aortic valve. There is also diastolic-spectral broadening characteristic of aortic regurgitation.

(b) The aortic systolic flow is approximately 2 m/second which is slightly increased and suggests the presence of mild aortic stenosis. Quantification of regurgitant lesions is more difficult; in regurgitation there is a jet of blood flowing from a high-pressure area into a low-pressure area. As a result there is a high-velocity laminar jet of flow in the regurgitant orifice itself, together with a flow disturbance in the chamber receiving the flow. To try to judge the severity a technique termed flow mapping is used. This requires pulsed Doppler. The sample-volume probe is sited in, and samples taken from, different regions of the appropriate chamber. This enables a picture to be built up of the spatial relationships of the regurgitant flow. If the flow disturbance is only present in the plane below the valve, then mild regurgitation is present; if the flow disturbance is distributed widely then severe regurgitation is present. The size of the chamber into which the jet flows will also have an influence on the flow characteristics.

(c) The introduction of color-flow Doppler enables more accurate estimation of the characteristics of flow.

91 (a) An AV-sequential or dual-chamber pacemaker.

(b) The pacemaker is responsive to the change in sinus rate associated with exercise. There is increasing evidence that in most patients, particularly younger patients, symptomatic state is better with an AV-sequential or dual-chamber pacemaker than with a ventricular pacemaker.

(c) It is technically more difficult to insert. It is more likely to malfunction than the simpler ventricular pacemaker. It is more expensive.

92 (a) Sinus rhythm with a normal PR interval. Left axis deviation. Right bundle branch block. Old lateral infarct. Old inferior infarct.

(b) The development of complete AV block and asystole.

(c) Insertion of a pacemaker.

93 (a) No. There is evidence of left atrial hypertension and right ventricular conduction delay.

(b) An echocardiogram might give valuable noninvasive information about the state of her myocardium.

(c) She had heart failure due to ischemic heart disease. Introduction of an ACE inhibitor caused the ECG changes of left atrial hypertension and conduction delay to improve.

94 (a) The right atrial pressure is grossly elevated. There is a very sharp Y descent and a moderately sharp X descent.

(b) Constrictive pericarditis.

(c) Both ventricles are constricted by the pericardium. The hemodynamic consequences are therefore equal for both ventricles, in contrast to heart failure where the left and right ventricular-function curves are no longer parallel.

95 (a) Loud first heart sound; systolic murmur; opening snap.

(b) She has mitral valve disease.

(c) The accurate timing of clicks and snaps. In most other ways the well-trained human ear is superior.

96 (a) The left atrium is very large. The enlargement may be because of the raised pressure in the left atrium; it is perhaps more likely to be the result of left myocardial involvement by rheumatic fever.

(b) The mitral valve. The reduced amplitude of excursion, the reduced diastolic closure rate, and the anterior movement of the posterior leaflet are due to the fibrosis, thickening, tethering, and commissural fusion that occur as a result of the rheumatic process.

(c) Yes. The interventricular septum does not move normally. This is because of the splinting effect of the rigid mitral valve.

97 (a) The left atrium is large; there is splaying of the carinal angle, there is the bulge on the left heart border, and there is a double density shadow to the right of the vertebral column. It is much more difficult to be certain about other chamber enlargement. The right atrium may be enlarged but it could just be pushed across by the left atrium. One of the ventricles is likely to be enlarged; on the basis that the clinical details are known, it is possible to deduce which one. Without the clinical details one cannot tell on the PA film and there is difficulty even with the help of a lateral.

(b) Upper-lobe blood diversion gives information on the left atrial pressure; if it is present, the left atrial pressure is likely to be at least 18 mmHg. Septal lines also indicate an elevated left atrial pressure.

98 (a) She has a marked scoliosis. This makes the interpretation of the heart's shape and size difficult. However, she does have a large heart. Both the pulmonary artery and left atrium appear to be large. It is difficult to see the pulmonary veins. The large heart suggests either a volume load on the ventricle or a myocardial problem.

(b) The combination of a large heart and prominent left atrium are indicative of mitral valve disease or a left ventricular myocardial problem.

99 (a) On the PA film the heart shadow may appear large.

(b) A systolic murmur may be found together with delayed closure of the pulmonary valve.

(c) Right bundle branch may be found.

100 (a) A large heart. There is also a fat pad which makes the heart appear even bigger. There is no evidence of a raised left atrial pressure.

(b) On the information given, it seems likely that he has an infection or perhaps a malignant process. The combination of a high venous pressure in someone who is comfortable lying flat raises the possibility of pericardial constriction.

(c) An echocardiogram will confirm the presence of pericardial fluid; it will not help determine the hemodynamic consequences of this fluid. A lateral X-ray of the chest can indirectly contribute to the diagnosis of pericardial fluid by inspection of the fat pad. Appropriate investigations will need to be performed to diagnose tuberculosis; pericardial aspiration is unfortunately often unhelpful in this regard.

101 (a) Bilateral flare from the hila. This is very suggestive of acute left ventricular failure.

(b) A rapid onset of shortness of breath suggests a number of possibilities; however, most of them would assume some prior underlying problem which was apparently absent in this man. A silent, acute infarct could present in this way but he is rather young for this. A ruptured chorda could account for this picture; pre-existing mitral valve disease would be likely. If there had been a history of chest trauma, an acute valve problem could have resulted. An arrhythmia superimposed on impaired left ventricular function would be a possibility if he had not been previously fit. An acute myocarditis is unlikely to present so dramatically. A myocardial toxin might cause such a presentation; cobalt, used to make beers more frothy, can present this acutely. Other toxins include scorpion venom, poisoning with phosphorus or arsenic, and drugs such as doxorubicin. The heart may be affected in anaphylaxis induced by drug sensitivity and can present in this way.

(c) The patient should respond to standard treatment for heart failure unless there is some irreversible process such as described above.

(d) A condition that must not be overlooked, since it is so easily treated, is thiamine deficiency. It can present acutely like this and may be made worse if you are keeping a vein open with a dextrose infusion.

ANSWERS

102 (a) The right ventricular diastolic pressure is identical with the left. Both diastolic pressures are elevated.

(b) The constricting force of the pericardium is equal for both ventricles and impairs ventricular filling.

(c) The cause of the shortness of breath in this setting is debatable but it probably relates to an inability of the cardiac output to rise appropriately with exertion; the shortness of breath is centrally mediated.

103 (a) Left coronary artery.

(b) The left main stem divides into anterior descending, and circumflex. The branches of the anterior descending include septal branches and, diagonal branch(es). The branches of the circumflex include the marginal branches, posterior left ventricular branches and, in some patients, the posterior descending branch and the branch to the AV node.

(c) Yes. The anterior descending supplies the proximal bundle branches and the bundle of His. In 20% of people the circumflex gives rise to the AV nodal branch.

(d) Yes. The anterior two-thirds is supplied by the anterior descending; in the 20% whose circumflex gives rise to the posterior descending, the posterior third of the septum will be supplied by this branch.

104 (a) A very large heart. There is no evidence of a raised left atrial pressure.

(b) A pericardial effusion. The etiology is difficult to predict without more clinical information.

(c) Sometimes the pericardial effusion can cause tamponade. This needs to be treated as a medical emergency with aspiration of fluid.

105 (a) The failing heart is less able to cope with varying ventricular rates than the normal heart. It is important to ensure that the ventricular rate is well controlled at all times.

(b) In the normal person one would expect the heart rate to be faster at certain times of the day and slower at others. The degree of variation in this patient is satisfactory for him, but would be unusual for a normal person.

(c) This is always a balanced decision. Undoubtedly his ventricular function would be helped by having sinus rhythm back again. The likelihood, however, of keeping him in sinus rhythm is small if his atrial fibrillation is long-standing. The addition of drugs, such as amiodarone, may increase the likelihood of him remaining in sinus rhythm but will adversely affect LV function.

106 (a) The aortic valve. The fact that it is difficult to see in the PA film means that it is overlying the vertebral column. If it were in any other valve position it would be to the side of the vertebral column and therefore more easily seen.

(b) Some models of the SE valve last for ever and outlive the patient. In most patients this valve will last in excess of 15 years.

(c) The mortality rate is about 1% per annum. The morbidity is considerably higher. Anticoagulation is also an inconvenience for the patient and adversely affects the quality of life.

107 (a) No. The relationship of the P wave to the QRS complex is inconsistent. This is AV dissociation but with a reasonable ventricular rate.

(b) It is likely that a 24-hour tape would show variation in the ventricular rate relating to the AV dissociation. This is usually a benign arrhythmia and the tape is unlikely to help therapeutically.

(c) A 24-hour tape involves a technician for about 10 minutes in setting up the tape and about 15 minutes in interpreting it. Doctor time is probably in the order of 5 minutes. The price, as opposed to the cost, seems to vary in the UK between £95 and £250. The actual cost is probably about £100 (1996 prices). This does not include the cost to the patient.

108 (a) Findings are compatible with moderately severe, reversible myocardial ischemia in the anteroseptal regions and inferior walls.

(b) Thallium is taken up only by nonischemic tissue. Exercise is performed and the image is obtained immediately after the stress of exercise. The delayed images are recorded several hours later when any residual myocardial ischemia should have resolved. The difference between the two images provides valuable information.

(c) The psychological impact of life in a city is considerable. There is much more stress associated with city life than rural life! It is not uncommon for patients to notice markedly different exercise tolerance in different situations; angina is not a 'free-standing entity' related just to coronary arteriographic findings!

109 (a) A narrow complex tachycardia with a ventricular rate of 206/minute.

(b) There are several clinical clues which can be helpful. These include:
(i) carotid-sinus massage which, if this were a supraventricular arrhythmia, would cause a sudden slowing of ventricular rate; (ii) listening to the first heart sound (if this were supraventricular tachycardia the first heart sound would be of constant intensity); if it were ventricular tachycardia then this would vary in intensity); (iii) the JVP may be helpful (if it were junctional tachycardia then fast cannon waves, at a rate of 206/minute, would be apparent; if it were ventricular tachycardia, irregular cannon waves would be apparent).

(c) This depends on the hemodynamic situation of the patient. If he is not hemodynamically compromised then a fairly leisurely approach can be adopted; this might include the use of (i) adenosine, or (ii) esmolol. These measures may diagnose the arrhythmia rather than cause persisting reversion to sinus rhythm. Secondly, intravenous verapamil might be used, provided that LV function is known to be good. If in doubt, verapamil should not be used. If the patient is hemodynamically compromised then a DC version is probably the treatment of choice.

110 (a) It is very abnormal. Only a very small part of the ventricle has a good amplitude of movement.

(b) No. There is a large segment of the left ventricle which is not in phase.

(c) This is very low.

(d) The ejection fraction of the contracting segment (CS EF) is shown to be 32%. This raises the possibility that, by removing the LV aneurysm, the remaining left ventricle may cope better; indeed, it may improve the overall function of the left ventricle and improve the symptoms of the patient.

111 (a) Gout is the likeliest diagnosis in the context of the presentation and treatment of heart failure.

(b) The acute attack is probably best managed with colchicine; this does not adversely affect the warfarin control. To introduce a nonsteroidal anti-inflammatory drug, particularly phenylbutazone, would radically change his anticoagulant control. In the longer term, allopurinol should be introduced to minimize the likelihood of further attacks.

112, 113

(a) The PA chest X-rays show a massively dilated and tortuous descending thoracic aorta. The sternal wires from the previous operation are present. The heart size itself is large.

(b) The major anxiety in this type of major operation to the thoracic aorta is that of a paraplegia; even in the best hands the risk of this is in the order of 5–8% and the mortality rate is about 15%.

(c) Control of any systemic hypertension is vital. The use of a beta-blocking drug is also valuable in order to reduce the shearing force on the vessel wall.

(d) Atherosclerosis is the most likely to condition to affect the aorta in this way. Other conditions to be considered would be: (i) syphilis (this usually affects the ascending aorta); (ii) cystic medical necrosis (this also usually affects the ascending aorta); (iii) a dissection (this can affect the descending aorta and spare the ascending aorta; it may be associated with (ii)).

114 (a) The diastolic pressures in the two ventricles are raised and are very similar; the two atrial pressures are similar and both are raised; the right ventricular and pulmonary artery systolic pressures are raised.

(b) The similar filling pressures of the two ventricles are very suggestive of constrictive pericarditis. If there were a left ventricular problem only, the LV diastolic pressure would be elevated more than the RV, which might be normal. A restrictive cardiomyopathy might produce this pattern but, again, one would expect some differentiation in the pressures between the right and left side of the heart.

(c) She had a constrictive pericarditis; surgical removal is the treatment of choice.

(d) The constriction of the pericardium affects both ventricles and atria; the hemodynamics are thus very different to those which pertain to left ventricular disease. In the latter, the very different right- and left-ventricular function curves cause the symptom of orthopnea.

115 (a) There is a very severe pressure difference between the right ventricle and the pulmonary artery. This pulmonary stenosis may be at valve level, sub-valve level or both.

(b) She will have an abnormal jugular venous pulse (JVP) with a dominant 'a' wave. The JVP may not be elevated. There will be RV hypertrophy manifest by a parasternal heave. There will be a systolic murmur, maximal in the pulmonary area, which will not radiate to the neck; it will not be a pansystolic murmur; it may be associated with a thrill. If the obstruction is at valve level there may be an ejection click. The second heart sound will be abnormal; P2 may be delayed or absent.

(c) She probably had a paradoxical embolism.

(d) On exertion her right atrial pressure will exceed her left atrial pressure; right-to-left shunting then takes place through an atrial-septal defect or a patent foramen ovale.

116 (a) This is a Dotter basket catheter.

(b) It has been introduced in order to snare and then remove the remains of a central venous catheter which has floated into the right ventricle.

117 (a) This is a normal ECG.

(b) If there is no historic lead, or an abnormality on examination, routine ECGs are unhelpful. Indeed, they can be positively dangerous in that they induce a false sense of security. The argument that they are useful in hindsight should something happen is weak, and does not help with the acute management of any presenting problem.

118 (a) Ankylosing spondylitis.

(b) Aortic regurgitation due to an associated aortitis.

(c) There is a long PR interval in association with aortic regurgitation. This relates to the inflammatory process spreading down to involve the conduction system.

119 (a) Large left ventricular cavity; poor movement of LV walls; small pericardial effusion; late opening of mitral valve; poor movement of aortic root; cusps of aortic valve float together during systole; slightly large left atrium.

(b) This appearance could be caused by a congestive cardiomyopathy; the pathology would be very nonspecific. It might be secondary to a myocarditis; if there was still an active inflammatory process, then there might be an inflammatory-cell infiltrate together with the fibrotic scarring. It might be caused by coronary artery disease.

(c) The heart murmur will be due to mitral or tricuspid regurgitation secondary to the dilatation of the left or right ventricles.

120 (a) The ECG shows a normal pacemaker artefact and normal pacing from the right ventricle.

(b) Yes. He will have reversed splitting of his second heart sound; he effectively has a left bundle branch block.

121 (a) Widespread hemorrhages. There are no obvious hypertensive changes. There is no papilledema.

b) Central retinal vein occlusion.

(c) Hypertension. Hematological abnormalities which increase the viscosity of the blood.

122 (a) Sinus bradycardia with well-marked U waves seen particularly in the left precordial leads and standard lead II leads. His serum potassium was 2.2 mmol/l.

(b) Potassium, either in dilute form intravenously or in tablet form. You will also need to think in terms of a potassium-conserving drug.

(c) Bananas and oranges contain high levels of potassium. These are not associated with some of the problems that occur with tablets.

123 (a) Sinus rhythm with evidence of an anterior myocardial infarct; the timing of the latter is difficult but it could have occurred 2 weeks ago.

(b) The operation should be postponed. The risk of surgery after a recent myocardial infarction is high; this risk remains for some 12 weeks and the operation should, if possible, be deferred until after this period has elapsed.

124 (a) The ECG is normal apart from a right bundle branch block. The complexes are all of a rather small voltage.

(b) A right bundle branch block can be a normal finding; the low voltage may be on the basis of her being overweight. If you think that her heart is normal then she can continue to hold the PSV licence. If there is any doubt in your mind, then further investigations need to be performed to clarify the situation.

125 (a) Wide splitting of the second heart sound; early systolic murmur; a right bundle branch block on the ECG. There is some AC (Alternating Current) interference on the ECG. The baseline is not very satisfactory in diastole; the appearance just before the first heart sound is caused by tricuspid closure and there is no diastolic murmur.

(b) An atrial-septal defect. It is difficult with the amount of information given to be certain that the second heart sound is relatively fixed in its splitting. The second component of the split sound is not an opening snap; you can identify the aortic closure because it occurs just before the dichrotic notch on the pulse tracing. The sound after the notch must therefore be pulmonary closure.

(c) If the shunt through the atrial-septal defect were large, a tricuspid flow murmur would be expected.

126 (a) The right ventricle may be large. The movement of the interventricular septum may move in an abnormal and paradoxical fashion; this allows the large RV volume to be accommodated. In the four-chamber view the interatrial septum may be visualized; if the atrial-septal defect is large then it may be visualized. If saline or dextrose is injected into a peripheral vein the microbubbles will be visualized as they pass through the right atrium and the right ventricle; they do not appear on the left side normally since they are 'filtered' by the lungs. In an atrial-septal defect there will be some right-to-left shunting and the microbubbles will be seen to pass from the right atrium to the left atrium.

(b) It is a superior investigation because: (i) better anatomic information is obtained; (ii) it is an easier technique to learn and on which to obtain reliable information; (iii) in conjunction with Doppler studies it will give both the anatomic information and also information about blood flow and velocity of flow; the echo is used to direct the Doppler beam to the point of interest.

(c) The value of the 2-D image is best appreciated on videotape recordings where the moving image is recorded. Still frames, for reproduction, lose a lot of their quality; this does not apply for the M-mode.

127 (a) Sinus rhythm with a normal PR interval; the QRS axis is posteriorly orientated; there is a dominant R wave in V1 and S waves in V5 and V6. These changes suggest right ventricular hypertrophy.

(b) There is no mention of any cyanosis and therefore a right-to-left shunt is unlikely; to present with syncope suggests the presence of pulmonary vascular disease. Nevertheless, knowledge of the size of the proximal pulmonary arteries would be of value. Radiologic evidence of lung disease or evidence of pulmonary emboli should be sought. Even though there is no diastolic murmur, evidence of a raised left atrial pressure should be sought.

(c) Was she taking the oral contraceptive pill? Had she been taking any slimming remedies?

(d) The pulmonary artery pressure could be measured; the absence of any shunt can be confirmed and the left atrial pressure shown to be normal. The pulmonary vascular resistance can then be calculated.

128 (a) Raised pulmonary artery pressure; raised right ventricular systolic and diastolic pressures; large 'a' wave in RA trace.

(b) Primary pulmonary hypertension. Thromboembolic pulmonary hypertension. Pulmonary hypertension due to high altitude or lung disease is unlikely, owing to the extreme level of the pulmonary artery pressure.

(c) High concentrations of oxygen are only of temporary value. Certain vasodilators such as nifedipine or the angiotensin-converting-enzyme (ACE) inhibitors may have a role which is occasionally dramatic. If a precipitating factor can be identified then it should be removed. Heart and lung transplantation is available for those patients who do not respond to these measures and who are suitable in other ways.

129 (a) Acute anterior infarction. Acute inferior infarction.

(b) Intravenous thrombolysis may cause the ECG to revert to normality; however, in this setting the changes are so widespread that complete reversion is unlikely.

(c) There is some evidence that acute coronary artery angioplasty may be a preferred option in patients with large infarctions; no appropriate trials comparing the two have yet been done. The time window for this to be achieved is relatively short.

130 (a) The picture shows an occluding thrombus in a coronary artery.

(b) It is now recognized that, in a large proportion of patients, the formation of an intraluminal thrombus plays an important part in a myocardial infarction. The rupture of the fibrous cap covering the atheromatous plaque allows the passage of blood into the intima with the formation of a thrombus and resulting in expansion of the plaque. There is also the development of a thrombus within the lumen; this does not necessarily occlude the lumen but initially waxes and wanes in size. If the thrombus occludes the vessel for long enough, a myocardial infarction ensues.

(c) Yes. The use of both aspirin and a fibrinolytic drug are of proven benefit as long as they are used within a few hours of the occlusion.

131 (a) The top recording shows a fast heart rate of 180/minute. The bottom recording shows sinus rhythm with a short PR interval and a heart rate of 47/minute. The fast rate is too fast to be a sinus tachycardia and is almost certainly an atrial tachycardia.

(b) Induction of retching; the Valsalva maneuver; swallowing of cold ice cream. Eyeball pressure should not be advised as retinal detachment has been reported. Carotid-sinus massage is actually very difficult for the patient to do.

(c) Often able to use intermittent drug therapy rather than continuous. The choice is large and will include a beta-blocker, verapamil, or amiodarone.

132 (a) Normal.

(b) Adenosine will vasodilate those vessels that are not diseased sufficiently to cause ischemia, i.e. that have the capacity to dilate. It acts as a sort of 'steal' and will expose the potentially ischemic zones.

(c) It will depend on the pre-test likelihood. In a UK hospital population it is likely to be in the order of a sensitivity of 0.85 and a specificity of 0.90.

133 (a) Paget's disease of bone.

(b) If a considerable proportion of the skeleton is involved, an increased cardiac output and increased pulse-pressure may occur. This is related to the multiple, small arteriovenous fistulae. A heart murmur due to the increased flow may therefore occur.

(c) Atrioventricular block may sometimes be associated with this condition, as can cor pulmonale.

134 (a) High end-diastolic pressure in left ventricle. Marked variation in systolic pressure in the presence of a sinus tachycardia.

(b) He has acute tamponade with a paradoxical pulse. It is likely that he sustained an aortic dissection.

(c) The pericardium is attached to the great vessels well above the aortic valve. The intimal tear in the aorta can enable blood to track down in the false lumen to below this pericardial attachment and blood will thus enter the pericardial space.

135 (a) Yes.

(b) Yes. The aorta overrides the interventricular septum; this is best seen in the top left tracing. Normally, the anterior wall of the aorta is continuous with the septum. In this patient, the septum appears to end in the center of the aorta; this is the overriding aorta.

(c) Tetralogy of Fallot.

ANSWERS

136 (a) In the left ventricle.

(b) The catheter has passed from IVC->->RA->->LA->->LV. The passage through the interatrial septum is either through a patent foramen ovale or through an atrial-septal defect.

(c) About 30% of normal people have a patent foramen ovale. In theory, therefore, this passage of the catheter can occur.

137 (a) Widespread bilateral shadowing of the lung fields.

(b) Pulmonary tuberculosis is the likeliest.

(c) The effects of sepsis. He may well have a reduced circulating volume and this might respond to rehydration. Early treatment of the underlying condition is essential. If this is proven to be tuberculosis, the prognosis is not good.

138 (a) There must be a communication between the aortic root and sternum. The sternum was eroded by the aorta.

(b) The aorta must communicate with another chamber as well as eroding the sternum.

(c) Syphilis. In fact he had high titers suggestive of active and recent disease.

139 (a) Very high chylomicron levels. The patient has a rare deficiency of lipoprotein lipase which is inherited on an autosomal recessive basis. The triglyceride levels are also elevated.

(b) Because the serum is clear, one can assume that the triglyceride levels are normal. The serum cholesterol is elevated.

(c) Since the serum is opalescent, one can assume that the triglyceride levels are elevated. No deduction can be made about the cholesterol level which may be high, low, or normal.

140 (a) He has a normal sized heart. The arch of the aorta is abnormal; the shape is characteristic of someone with a coarctation showing the reversed-3 sign. There is well-shown rib notching.

(b) There may be an associated bicuspid aortic valve. Congenital berry aneurysms are also associated.

(c) In this condition there is often a typical marked tortuosity of the arterioles.

(d) The blood pressure may rise steeply.

141 (a) A large bulge on the left heart border which represents an LV aneurysm.

(b) Heart failure; arrhythmias; emboli; rupture.

(c) Echocardiogram (ideally two-dimensional); radio-isotope studies; angiography; fluoroscopy; clinical examination.

142 (a) Long PR interval (first-degree AV block); voltage criteria of left ventricular hypertrophy.

(b) The combination of aortic regurgitation and a long PR interval is suggestive of an aortitis, such as ankylosing spondylitis or Reiter's syndrome.

(c) In these conditions the inflammatory process and adventitial thickening spreads down from the aorta to involve the membranous ventricular septum and the base of the mitral valve. It can therefore involve the conducting system.

(d) Manifestations of the arthropathy, eye changes, etc.

(e) A high proportion of individuals afflicted have the HLA-B27 antigen.

143 (a) The right atrial pressure is high.

(b) The right-sided saturations are all a little low. There is arterial desaturation related to a right-to-left shunt at atrial level.

(c) There is an obstruction at the tricuspid valve level; this could be a tumor or thrombus. There might be disease of the tricuspid valve, but there are no supportive clues due to the patient's short history.

144 (a) The echocardiogram is normal. You need to see the video in order to give a proper report.

(b) There is no evidence of endocarditis. However, the echocardiogram cannot rule out the possibility of the diagnosis, which has to be made on other criteria.

145 (a) It shows atrial flutter with 2:1 conduction. There are Q waves in V1 and V2. There is poor R-wave progression.

(b) He needs to be converted out of atrial flutter. This could be achieved either by DC shock or by chemical means. Digoxin is likely to convert atrial flutter to atrial fibrillation.It is alleged that stopping digoxin then causes reversion to sinus rhythm.

(c) Warfarin needs to be considered because of the risk of thromboembolism. Although atrial flutter has a theoretically smaller likelihood than atrial fibrillation, in a patient in this age group who has heart failure the risk is real and could be reduced by warfarin.

146 (a) Sinus bradycardia; J waves; long QT interval.

(b) Hypothermia.

(c) Reduced intake while becoming hypothermic; polyuria due to tubular dysfunction in hypothermia; rewarming producing vasodilatation.

147 (a) She is having a balloon mitral valvuloplasty. The balloon being used is an Innoue balloon.

(b) The balloon is sited in the left atrium. It is introduced through the left atrium in a deflated and extended state so that its circumference is minimized. It is introduced through the interatrial septum. It is then positioned across the mitral valve and inflated to a pre-set diameter.

(c) Embolization is the most worrying complication. Most centers now do both transthoracic and transesophageal echoes to exclude clot. Moreover, the patient is anticoagulated for several weeks before the procedure. Less common problems relate to acute tamponade caused by perforation of the atrial wall, arrhythmias, and the development of pulmonary edema during inflation.

148 (a) There are two leads, one to the atrium and one to the ventricles. This is a dual-chamber pacemaker.

(b) The aortic valve is calcified. It is likely therefore that she has aortic valve disease; she may also have other valve disease.

(c) Calcification in and around the aortic annulus will often involve the conducting system. The bundle of His is only 1–2 mm away from the aortic annulus.

149 (a) The ascending aorta and the descending aorta have an intimal flap demonstrated; this results from a dissection of the aorta.

(b) The left atrium.

(c) Pulmonary veins.

(d) The descending aorta.

150 (a) An enlarged heart. The lung fields look normal.

(b) He may have underlying heart muscle disease.

(c) He may be HIV positive; he will thus be predisposed to infections which may make endocarditis more likely. There is also some evidence that, in the absence of infections, heart muscle disease occurs in these patients; this may be on an immunologic basis.

151 (a) A large heart; large proximal pulmonary arteries; no peripheral 'pruning' of pulmonary vessels.

(b) A left-to-right shunt. The level is difficult to determine without more information. The most likely shunt at this age would be an atrial-septal defect.

(c) There is a large shunt as manifest by the size of the pulmonary vessels. Surgical correction of the shunt is the preferred treatment.

(d) If there were to be a high pulmonary vascular resistance, then surgery would be contraindicated. This seems unlikely in this case because of the lack of pruning.

152 (a) There is some confluent shadowing in the right, middle, and lower zones of the lung.

(b) The tip of the nasogastric tube is seen in the right lower-lobe bronchus; the enteral feeding fluid has entered the lung, causing the radiographic changes and her symptoms.

(c) Removal of the nasogastric tube and energetic physiotherapy.

153 (a) Enlarged heart; large left atrium; some shadowing at the left base.

(b) The left atrium which is extremely large.

(c) Rheumatic heart disease.

(d) A heterograft or xenograft; this is tissue from another animal species (the usual one used is a pig). A homograft or valve from the same animal species. An autograft or valve from the same person; the valve from another site can be switched. A prosthetic or man-made valve; there are a variety of designs and makes of these.

154, 155

(a) There is an enlarged left atrium. The heart size is normal. There is upper-lobe blood diversion.

(b) The left atrium is enlarged. There is no valve calcification.

(c) With an enlarged left atrium there is a risk that certain types of medication may be held up in the esophagus and cause local damage; this particularly applies to slow-release potassium chloride tablets. The only other gut problem is, of course, embolism to the gut arteries.

(d) The temptation to anticoagulate the patient immediately must be resisted. The risk of anticoagulation, and thus of causing bleeding into the ischemic brain, is high and is present regardless of whether the initial event was thrombotic, embolic, or a hemorrhage. Although this opinion is somewhat controversial, the author recommends that the interval between the event and the initiation of anticoagulation should be at least 4 weeks.

156 (a) The left ventricular systolic pressure is high. The left ventricular diastolic pressure is high. The systolic pressure alternates between high and low pressure.

(b) The ventricular equivalent of pulsus alternans signifies a ventricle that is failing. She is in urgent need of aortic valve replacement.

(c) She is very unlikely to be alive at the end of 1 year unless the obstructed aortic valve has been rectified surgically.

157 (a) Asystole. The asystole involves the sinus node, atria, and ventricles. There is a long pause associated with no cardiac output.

(b) She will require permanent pacing.

(c) Yes. She is at high risk of death and needs to be monitored until the permanent pacemaker is inserted; if this is going to be delayed, then a temporary wire ought to be inserted.

158 (a) First-degree heart block; partial right bundle branch block; left axis deviation with left anterior hemi-block.

(b) Development of complete AV block with associated episodes of asystole or ventricular fibrillation.

(c) Insertion of permanent pacemaker.

159 (a) This is a multiple-gated acquisition (MUGA) scan.

(b) The principle of the scan is to use the R wave of the ECG as the triggering signal. The radionuclide data from the injected radio-isotope is collected and segregated temporarily into 16–28 equal divisions or pixels, depending on the heart rate. Studies require from 2 to 10 minutes for completion. A left and right ventricular time–activity curve is based on analysis of the left anterior oblique position. To obtain information about regional wall movement, several different views are required.

(c) Atrial fibrillation or frequent and persistent ectopic activity make the study virtually impossible. The inability of the patient to lie still also makes the study difficult.

(d) There are several circumstances in which this investigation can give useful information. In the patient being considered for surgery, an accurate estimate of their ejection fraction will aid the decision-making process. In the patient with an aneurysm, this study will give a good estimate of the function of the remaining LV.

(e) This scan shows generally very poor ventricular function. The amplitude image shows poor amplitude of left ventricular wall motion. The phase image is extremely fragmented, demonstrating discoordinate ventricular contraction. The ejection fraction of each ventricle is in the order of 6–8%. If an operation were being contemplated, the chances of getting him off the operating table would be very low.

160 (a) By constructing volume curves throughout the cardiac cycle from each pixel of a gated blood-pool scan, color-coded images of amplitude of regional wall motion, and phase of wall motion can be generated. In this example the normal-phase image shows that both ventricles contract uniformly and in synchrony (coded green); the atria (coded red) are 180° out of phase. The amplitude image shows vigorous LV contraction.

(b) Yes.

(c) It is a normal study.

161 (a) The rhythm is a junctional one.

(b) At the bedside you should be able to see regular cannon waves.

(c) The esophageal lead enables you to identify the atrial activity if it is hidden within the ventricular complexes on the surface ECG. Having identified the atrial activity, it is then possible to determine its relationship to the ventricular complexes. If you know the siting of the tip of the esophageal lead (distance from the mouth) then you can, from the shape or vectors of the atrial complexes, determine the origin of the rhythm in the atria.

162 (a) An atrial rhythm; atrial and ventricular asystole; sinus rhythm.

(b) This patient has sinoatrial disease and ventricular conducting-system disease. In the light of the symptoms a pacemaker is the preferred treatment.

(c) Conducting tissue disease can be part of a chronic fibrotic process of unknown etiology. Although it is often associated with coronary artery disease, there is little evidence to demonstrate a cause-and-effect relationship. In certain parts of the world it can be part of a systemic disease such as Chagas' disease.

163 (a) There is a marked inflammatory response with infiltrates of white cells. There is some destruction of muscle fibers and some early fibrotic changes.

(b) The picture is one of a myocarditis; the most likely etiology is viral. The commonest viral agents are a coxsackie B or echovirus.

(c) A myocarditis is a very common complication of any systemic viral illness such as influenza; the vast majority of people recover without sequelae. A small number will go on to develop heart failure and a small group will present with sudden death.

(d) It is very important that energetic exercise is avoided during the weeks following the infection. All too often it is a premature return to strenuous activity that precipitates a demise.

164 (a) The patient has dextrocardia. The pattern differs from incorrect lead attachments inasmuch as V4R and V5R have progressively increasing R waves and V4 and V5 have progressively decreasing R waves.

(b) The patient might have Kartagener's syndrome which is associated with sinusitis, dextrocardia, and oligospermia or infertility.

(c) The infertility or oligospermia and the sinusitis are related to malfunction of cilia. The structural abnormality can be seen on electron microscopy. Specific defects include defects in the dynein arms, spokes, or microtubule doublets. Cilia from epithelia and sperm tails, from the same individual, exhibit the same defects.

165 (a) No. There is a short PR interval and delta waves. The patient has Wolff–Parkinson–White syndrome (WPW).

(b) Reciprocating atrial tachycardia. Alternatively, he may develop atrial fibrillation; this is a very serious condition when associated with WPW.

(c) Electrophysiological studies to identify an accessory pathway and, if possible, to ablate it.

166 (a) Extremely thick interventricular septum; systolic anterior movement of the mitral valve; slow diastolic closure rate of the mitral valve; pericardial fluid.

(b) Hypertrophic obstructive cardiomyopathy together with a pericardial effusion.

(c) Typical. Angina is very common in severe forms of this condition. Dizziness or syncope after exercise is also typical and differs from the symptoms that occur with exertion in aortic valve stenosis.

(d) An arrhythmia. Anti-arrhythmic drug therapy.

(e) Yes. The condition may be inherited on a dominant basis.

ANSWERS

167, 168

(a) Coarctation of the aorta, in the classic position, just distal to the origin of the left subclavian.

(b) The hypertension in the upper arm is much easier to control after the coarctation has been operated upon.

(c) Brachial–femoral delay; a late systolic murmur best heard over the left scapula, which may spill over into diastole. There may be palpable collateral vessels with associated bruits.

(d) The triad consists of aortic valve disease, coarctation of the aorta, and berry aneurysm in the circle of Willis.

(e) Paraplegia.

169 (a) The heart is slightly large; the aortic knuckle is small; the pulmonary arteries to all zones of the lung are large (there is therefore pulmonary plethora); there is no pruning of the pulmonary arteries.

(b) A left-to-right shunt. We need the clinical information in order to be more precise. The small aortic knuckle is more suggestive of an atrial-septal defect than the other shunts.

(c) In order to get plethora the shunt has to have at least a pulmonary–systemic flow ratio of 2:1. This is severe enough to cause the development of pulmonary hypertension and reversal of the shunt.

(d) The shunt can be calculated by performing catheter studies and measuring saturations. Electrocardiography can also be used to estimate the size of shunt. It is likely that this particular shunt will work out to have a flow ratio of at least 2:1 and more likely 3:1. If the patient had presented at a younger age, surgery would have been advised. Some patients with a large shunt go through life without running into serious hemodynamic trouble.

170 (a) No. The PR interval on the first three beats of the top trace is varying and this is probably a slow idioventricular rhythm. The subsequent QRS complexes have an inverted P wave following them. These are junctional or high ventricular focus.

(b) She will have regular cannon waves during the arrhythmia; each atrial contraction is against a closed AV valve.

(c) If the symptoms are not troubling her unduly frequently, she is probably better off without any treatment. Any antiarrhythmic drug that is going to slow her inherent rate will probably not help.

171 (a) A very enlarged heart. The right-heart border suggests right atrial enlargement. The film is rather overexposed which makes comments about the vascular pattern in the lungs difficult.

(b) On a PA chest X-ray it is not possible to determine which of the ventricles is enlarged; it may be both. Even with the help of a lateral you will be wrong fairly frequently. Both atria are very large in this patient.

(c) Large atria 'accommodate' severe regurgitation much better than small chambers. As a result the patient remains less symptomatic for longer.

172 (a) Both the limb leads and the praecordial leads are suggestive of dextrocardia.
(b) The aortic area and pulmonary areas are transposed; it is actually A2 that is being heard.
(c) Ask the technician to record the ECG again with the arm leads transposed and the precordial leads recorded as V6R, V5R, V4R, etc.

173 (a) There is an extremely thick interventricular septum. The posterior LV wall is also thick. The aortic valve looks normal.
(b) Although there is hypertrophy of both the free LV wall and the IV septum, it is likely that the patient has hypertrophic cardiomyopathy which is probably obstructive.

174 (a) The long-axis view of the heart.
(b) Thick interventricular septum; echogenic myocardium; pericardial fluid; slightly thickened aortic valve.
(c) There may be an infiltrative process; examples might be amyloid or sarcoid. In this instance the patient had amyloid.

175 (a) A right-sided pneumothorax is present. There is shadowing at the right apex, at the right base, and hilum. The appearance of these shadows suggests an infective cause. The appearances in the lung suggest that some of the lesions may be cavitating.
(b) The appearances are consistent with embolic infected material causing lung abscesses; they raise the possibility of a right-sided endocarditis with perhaps a staphylococcus as the infecting organism.
(c) Right-sided endocarditis. The clinical diagnosis of a right-sided endocarditis is difficult. If the heart previously had been normal, there may be no murmurs. If the tricuspid valve is involved there will be none of the typical signs associated with chronic tricuspid valve disease; there will be no pulsatile liver and perhaps no murmurs. The only abnormal sign may be an abnormal character of the JVP. The diagnosis is made by first considering it. Careful examination of the JVP and careful auscultation may give a lead. Blood cultures are essential. An echocardiogram may demonstrate the vegetations, but their absence does not exclude the diagnosis.

176 (a) Fracture of the shaft of the femur with displacement.
(b) Probably related to fat emboli; this has a typical distribution around the upper part of the chest anteriorly and the neck.
(c) Blood gases. He is likely to be hypoxic, owing to the fat embolism, and requires supplemental oxygen.
(d) Fat emboli are remarkably common; long-bone fractures are not necessary to produce it. For the most part it is not recognized and the prognosis is good. However, the more severely affected patient, such as this one, can become very ill; the process can be complicated by disseminated intravascular coagulation and/or adult respiratory distress syndrome (ARDS).

ANSWERS

177 (a) Sinus rhythm with a long PR interval. There is a right bundle block pattern. There are very large P waves of right atrial hypertrophy.

(b) Her right atrial hypertrophy is gross. In the absence of good evidence of right ventricular hypertrophy the likely abnormality is Ebstein's anomaly. Although she could have right ventricular hypertrophy (and this might be difficult to interpret through a right-bundle branch block), there was no clinical evidence of it. During an arrhythmia the output falls dramatically, owing to the loss of atrial transport and the associated RV myopathy.

(c) Ebstein's anomaly is often associated with right-to-left shunting at the atrial level. There is often an associated cardiomyopathy affecting the right ventricle. With a rise in right atrial pressure during the arrhythmia, the degree of right-to-left shunting increases.

178 (a) Large heart; pleural calcification in both the left apex and right mid-zone.

(b) He had pulmonary tuberculosis. The large heart reflects his valvular disease.

179 (a) She has widespread surgical emphysema. She also has mediastinal emphysema.

(b) No. Conventional treatment for her asthma should suffice and the surgical emphysema will resolve.

(c) It is unusual but well recognized.

180 (a) Widespread surgical emphysema. There is also a pneumopericardium.

(b) A pneumopericardium can be associated with most unusual heart sounds which can sometimes be of a 'crunching' nature.

(c) No. The surgical emphysema and the pneumopericardium will resolve spontaneously.

181 (a) One is sited in the superior vena cava; it looks as though this is inserted through an infraclavicular subclavian route. There is also a Swan–Ganz catheter sited in the pulmonary artery and this has been inserted via the jugular vein.

(b) The right atrial pressure can be measured in the catheter sited in the superior vena cava. The pulmonary artery pressure can be measured with the Swan–Ganz catheter. By inflating the balloon, an indirect left atrial pressure can be recorded.

(c) In this setting of septicemia and ARDS, it is important to know about the filling pressures of both ventricles. The right atrial pressure and left atrial pressure give this information. Also, using the Swan–Ganz catheter, information can be gained about the systemic vascular resistance and cardiac output. Depending on the results of these calculations, drugs such as epinephrine, norepinephrine, or vasodilating agents can be used in order to optimize cardiac output, oxygen delivery, and the peripheral vascular resistance.

182 (a) The endotracheal tube down the right main bronchus; an opacifying left lung; the mediastinum shifting towards the left.

(b) The endotracheal tube needs to be pulled back so that it sits in the trachea rather than the bronchi. Also, this should allow the left lung to be ventilated adequately and the secretions to be cleared.

(c) The left side of the chest would not be moving as well as the right.

183 (a) Cardiomegaly; prominent ascending aorta; multiple bullae on the left side.

(b) The shape of the heart suggests aortic regurgitation or mixed aortic valve disease.

184 (a) Cardiomegaly. Pulmonary plethora; the pulmonary arteries to each zone of the lung are larger than normal. Calcification within a PDA.

(b) The left atrium and left ventricle have to cope with the volume load. The right ventricle is protected by the pulmonary valve. There is no additional load to the right ventricle until such time as pulmonary hypertension supervenes.

(c) Differential cyanosis when pulmonary hypertension and reversal of the shunt occurs. The cyanosis will be to the legs, but not to the arms, as long as the PDA inserts distal to the origin of the left subclavian artery.

185 (a) A burst of ultrasound is emitted by the transducer which then receives the signals from the depth of interest. The return signal is analyzed for Doppler shifts which correspond to the rate of blood flow. The rates are color-coded from orange to red to blue, reflecting faster to slower rates.

(b) An atrial-septal defect with a left-to-right shunt.

(c) She is likely to have a mid-systolic murmur arising from the outflow tract of the right ventricle, reflecting the increased volume of flow. She is likely to have fixed splitting of her second heart sound. She may also have a tricuspid diastolic flow murmur. The fixed splitting is related to the fact that the atria function as a common collecting chamber and that the respiratory variation of blood volume returning to the chambers of the heart is evened out. The delay in pulmonary closure reflects the increased volume and also often reflects an associated bundle branch block. The flow across the atrial septum is at low pressure and will not be audible.

186 (a) There is a solid mass in the subcarinal region, splaying the carinal angle and extending into the inferior left hemithorax, engulfing the left hilar structures. There is elevation of the left hemi-diaphragm.

(b) The left diaphragm is elevated and it is likely that the left phrenic nerve and left recurrent pharyngeal nerve are involved.

(c) Extensive bronchogenic carcinoma.

187 (a) Coarctation of the aorta with or without a bicuspid aortic valve.

(b) There is a normal tricuspid appearance to the aortic valve. There is no evidence of coarctation.

(c) Aneurysm in the circle of Willis. The triad is a bicuspid aortic valve, coarctation, and an aneurysm in the circle of Willis.

188 (a) A very dilated ascending aorta giving the appearance of gross widening of the mediastinum.

(b) The heart is very large and the walls look very thickened, owing to LV hypertrophy related to the hypertension.

189 (a) She has a ruptured aortic aneurysm and there is a lot of blood in the posterior part of the abdominal cavity on the left.

(b) Emergency surgery is her only hope.

(c) A pulsatile abdominal mass; this may be absent if her hemodynamic state has deteriorated too far.

190 (a) There is free blood in the left pleural space. The appearance of the descending aorta shows a true lumen and a false lumen.

(b) Acute aortic dissection with extravasation of the fluid into the left pleural space.

(c) He needs to be stabilized. His blood pressure needs to be brought down to a systolic of 100 mmHg. He needs to be started on a beta-blocker to slow the rate of rise of the arterial pulse. He has to have his pain relieved. Once stable he should be transferred to a cardiothoracic center where angiography should be performed. If it is a dissection involving the aortic root, then surgery would be advised.

191 (a) Papilledema with flame-shaped hemorrhages and exudates.

(b) Accelerated hypertension with papilledema and exudates. This used to be called 'malignant' hypertension because in the years before hypotensive drug-therapy it was associated with death within a relatively short period of time. Now with good control of blood pressure the prognosis is very much more satisfactory.

(c) Smooth lowering of his blood pressure and then careful monitoring of the blood pressure together with renal function. He will obviously need careful investigations to pursue any secondary cause.

192 (a) In the absence of trauma the sudden onset of a lesion of this nature suggests an inflammatory process, or perhaps a vasculitic one.

(b) In this setting, a blood culture would be the most important investigation. If a vasculitic process was likely, then an erythrocyte sedimentation rate measurement would be useful. Other investigations, such as white cell count and C-reactive protein, would also be high on the list.

193 (a) An area of calcification within the heart shadow.

(b) This is almost certainly a calcified ventricular aneurysm secondary to a previous myocardial infarction.

(c) If the patient is asymptomatic then the only measures that need to be addressed are the secondary prevention aspects. His cholesterol should be checked and brought down to < 4.2 mmol/l. His blood pressure will need to be assessed and treated if necessary. Advice about cigarette smoking should be given if he is a smoker. He should be taking aspirin on a regular basis.

194 (a) Transesophageal echocardiography is performed with a transducer positioned behind the heart in the esophagus. There is no intervening air such as with transthoracic echocardiography; the window therefore is much larger. The density of the intervening tissues is much less with TEE and the quality of the study is likely to be greater.

(b) TEE involves placing a relatively large transducer in the esophagus; there is a need, therefore, for the back of the throat and larynx to be anesthetized. It is a more uncomfortable procedure than transthoracic echocardiography but the quality of the images can be much better, particularly the structures at the back of the heart.

(c) Part of the circumference of the valve has become detached. As a result, in the doppler study, flow can be seen extending through the gap between the valve and the valve ring into the left atrium and right to the back of it the atrium. This is quite severe mitral regurgitation.

(d) Replacement of the valve.

195 (a) A mass within the left atrium.

(b) This is likely to be a left atrial myxoma. The systemic symptoms can mimic endocarditis and will resolve when the myxoma is removed.

(c) Surgical removal of the myxoma.

(d) The family should be screened as it can sometimes run in families.

196 (a) With an abnormal resting ECG an exercise-stress test on a treadmill cannot be interpreted with any degree of confidence.

(b) The stress images or delayed images show marked reduction of the tracer up-take in the apex and inferior walls; the redistribution or delayed images showed no change.

(c) It is now recognized that the myocardium, when ischemic, or following an infarction, can appear to be nonfunctional and dead. However, within the ischemic or apparent necrotic zones there is a viable myocardium which can function normally again when perfusion is restored.

197 (a) Very large proximal pulmonary arteries to each zone of the lung (i.e. plethora); calcification within the pulmonary arteries; rapid change in the caliber of the pulmonary arteries rather than a smooth tapering (i.e. pruning); large heart.

(b) A left-to-right shunt in which pulmonary arterial hypertension has developed. The development of cyanosis means that the shunt has now begun to reverse. The only lesion that produces such large pulmonary arteries and a large heart is an atrial-septal defect.

(c) There is now no place for surgery. Indeed, an operation might actually shorten her life. The treatment therefore is tailored for complications such as polycythemia or heart failure.

198 (a) Low pulmonary artery pressure; high infundibular pressure; very high pressure in the body of the right ventricle; pressure difference or gradient at valvular and infundibular levels.

(b) The patient probably has Fallot's tetralogy and the cyanosis is on the basis of right-to-left shunting at ventricular level.

(c) Squatting. This raises systemic resistance and thereby enhances pulmonary flow.

(d) Surgery. Both the valvular and infundibular obstructions can be relieved and the ventricular-septal defect closed. The patient will still have residual abnormalities in the right ventricular outflow tract and will continue to have a need for follow-up in a medical clinic. The patient should continue to take precautions for any septic procedures.

199 (a) The ECG is recorded at the wrong paper speed; in this instance it is recorded at 10 mm/second instead of 25 mm/second. There are abnormal T waves in V6. There are also voltage criteria of left ventricular hypertrophy.

(b) Repeat the ECG at a normal paper speed.

200 (a) The aortic valve is heavily calcified; it is difficult actually to see any orifice at all. In this view, one is looking into the aortic valve from above and normally would see it open widely in systole.

(b) The long-axis view shows the thickened, calcified aortic valve, and a normal sized LV cavity; the definition of the still frame is not good enough to determine the degree of hypertrophy of the LV walls; the left atrium is enlarged.

(c) She has severe aortic valve stenosis.

(d) The ECG may give some additional indirect evidence of the severity. The physical examination is, of course, the best noninvasive means of all. The Doppler/echocardiogram is an extremely useful investigation and can give good information about the severity of this valve lesion. The use of systolic time intervals can also give helpful information.

138